# THE ULTIMATE YOGA GUIDE FOR WOMEN

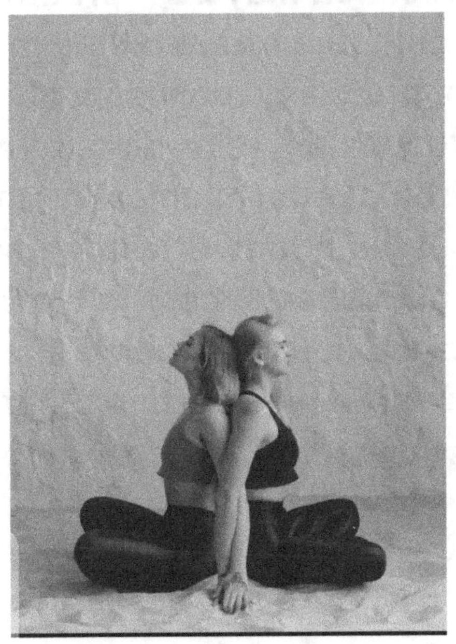

**"A Comprehensive Handbook for Women's Health and Well-being through Yoga"**

**EMMA LYNCH**

# TABLE OF CONTENTS

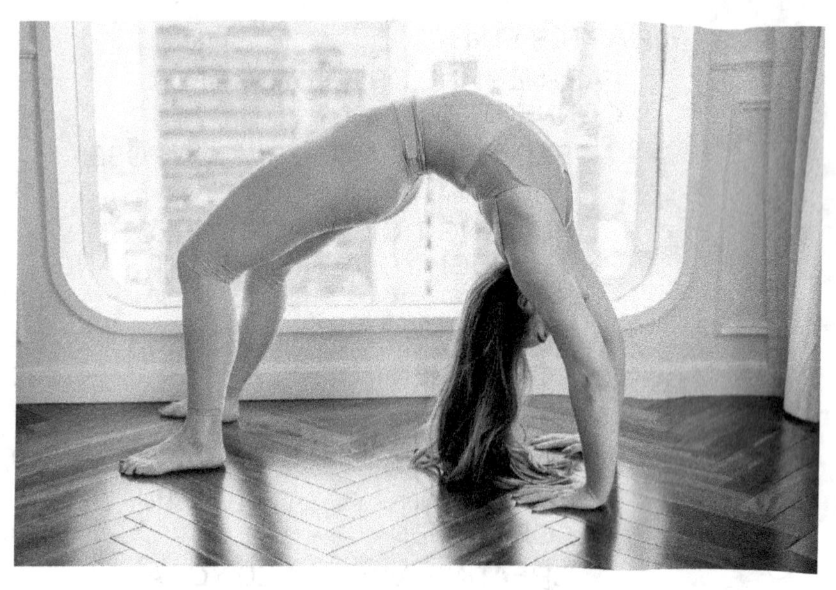

# INTRODUCTION TO YOGA FOR WOMEN

Yoga has emerged as a transformative practice that encompasses physical, mental, and spiritual dimensions, offering profound benefits tailored to women's unique needs and experiences. Rooted in ancient Indian tradition, yoga has evolved into a globally recognized system of holistic wellness, attracting millions of practitioners worldwide, including a significant number of women. In this introductory chapter, we delve into the essence of yoga for women, exploring its origins, principles, and the manifold ways it contributes to women's health and well-being.

Historically, yoga has been practiced predominantly by men, with ancient texts and scriptures often portraying male sages and ascetics as its primary proponents. However, as yoga spread beyond its cultural boundaries and gained popularity in modern society, women have increasingly embraced and shaped its practice. Today, women make up a substantial portion of yoga practitioners globally, drawn to its inclusive and adaptable nature, which resonates with their diverse lifestyles and needs.

At its core, yoga is more than just physical exercise; it is a holistic system that integrates body, mind, and spirit. Through a combination of physical postures (asanas), breathing techniques (pranayama), meditation, and ethical principles, yoga seeks to promote harmony and balance within oneself and with the surrounding world. For women, yoga offers a sanctuary—a space where they can nurture themselves, cultivate self-awareness, and foster inner strength amidst the myriad demands and pressures of daily life.

One of the key pillars of yoga for women is its emphasis on self-care and self-compassion. In a world that often imposes unrealistic standards and expectations on women's bodies and minds, yoga provides a refuge where women can reconnect with their innate wisdom and intuition, honoring their bodies' unique capabilities and limitations. Through gentle movement, conscious breathing, and mindfulness practices, women can cultivate a deeper sense of self-love and acceptance, fostering resilience and empowerment from within.

Moreover, yoga offers specific benefits tailored to women's health concerns across the lifespan. From supporting menstrual health and fertility to easing the transitions of pregnancy and menopause, yoga offers practical tools and techniques to navigate the intricate tapestry of women's reproductive and hormonal experiences. Additionally, yoga has been shown to alleviate stress, anxiety, and depression—common challenges that disproportionately affect women—providing a holistic approach to mental and emotional well-being.

In essence, yoga for women is not just a physical practice but a journey of self-discovery, healing, and empowerment. As women embrace the transformative potential of yoga, they embark on a path of profound personal growth and holistic wellness, enriching their lives and the lives of those around them. Through this guide, we invite women of all ages and backgrounds to embark on this empowering journey, unlocking the boundless potential that lies within each breath, each pose, and each moment of mindful awareness.

# WHY YOGA IS ESSENTIAL FOR WOMEN'S HEALTH

Yoga is essential for women's health due to its multifaceted approach to well-being, addressing physical, mental, and emotional aspects unique to women's experiences. Here's why yoga is indispensable for women's health:

1. **Physical Health Benefits**: Yoga offers a comprehensive workout that enhances flexibility, strength, and balance, promoting overall physical fitness. It targets specific areas of concern for women, such as pelvic floor muscles, core strength,

and joint mobility, thereby reducing the risk of injuries and promoting better posture.

2. **Menstrual Health and Hormonal Balance**: Certain yoga poses and breathing techniques are specifically designed to alleviate menstrual discomfort and regulate hormonal imbalances. Practices like restorative yoga and gentle twists can help relieve menstrual cramps, while pranayama techniques promote hormonal balance, reducing symptoms of PMS and menopause.

3. **Pregnancy and Postnatal Well-being**: Prenatal yoga offers numerous benefits for expectant mothers, including improved flexibility, strength, and relaxation, while also fostering a deeper connection with the unborn child. Postnatal yoga helps women regain strength and flexibility after childbirth, promotes faster recovery, and assists in relieving common postpartum discomforts.

4. **Emotional and Mental Health**: Yoga serves as a powerful tool for managing stress, anxiety, and depression, which disproportionately affect women. Mindfulness practices incorporated into yoga, such as meditation and deep breathing, help women cultivate inner peace, resilience, and emotional balance, empowering them to navigate life's challenges with greater ease.

5. **Bone Health and Osteoporosis Prevention**: Weight-bearing yoga poses help strengthen bones, reducing the risk of osteoporosis—a condition more prevalent in women. Regular practice of yoga postures that engage major muscle groups, such as standing poses and inversions, contributes to bone density and overall skeletal health.

6. **Heart Health and Blood Pressure Regulation**: Certain yoga practices, such as gentle flows and relaxation techniques, have been shown to lower blood pressure and improve cardiovascular health. Women, who often face increased risk of heart disease and hypertension, can benefit from incorporating yoga into their lifestyle to promote heart health and reduce the risk of cardiovascular complications.

7. **Self-Care and Empowerment**: Yoga encourages women to prioritize self-care and cultivate a compassionate relationship with their bodies. By honoring their physical and emotional needs on the mat, women learn to extend that same care and kindness to themselves in everyday life, fostering a sense of empowerment and self-love.

In summary, yoga plays a vital role in supporting women's health by addressing their unique physiological, psychological, and emotional needs. Its holistic approach promotes physical vitality, emotional resilience, and mental clarity, empowering women to lead healthier, happier lives at every stage of their journey.

# HOW YOGA BENEFITS WOMAN PHYSICALLY AND MENTALLY

Yoga offers a multitude of physical and mental benefits for women, contributing to their overall health and well-being in profound ways:

**Physical Benefits:**

1. **Flexibility:** Yoga incorporates a wide range of stretching and bending poses that improve flexibility, making it easier for women to move with ease in their daily activities. Enhanced flexibility also reduces the risk of injury and muscle strain.

2. **Strength:** Many yoga poses require women to engage and strengthen various muscle groups, including the core, arms, legs, and back. Regular practice builds muscular strength, contributing to better posture, balance, and overall physical strength.

3. **Balance and Coordination:** Yoga poses often involve balancing on one leg or holding positions that challenge coordination and proprioception. Over time, women develop better balance and coordination, which are essential for

stability and injury prevention, especially as they age.

4. **Joint Health:** Yoga promotes joint health by encouraging gentle movement through a full range of motion. Poses like lunges, twists, and backbends help lubricate the joints, reduce stiffness, and alleviate tension, promoting better joint function and mobility.

5. **Cardiovascular Health:** Certain yoga practices, such as dynamic flows and sequences, elevate the heart rate and increase blood circulation, improving cardiovascular health. Regular practice can lower blood pressure, reduce cholesterol levels, and enhance heart function, lowering the risk of heart disease.

**Mental Benefits:**

1. **Stress Reduction:** Yoga is renowned for its stress-relieving effects, as it encourages deep breathing, mindfulness, and relaxation. Women often face numerous stressors in their lives, and yoga provides a sanctuary where they can unwind, release tension, and restore inner peace.

2. **Anxiety and Depression Management:** Studies have shown that yoga can be effective in alleviating symptoms of anxiety and depression. Mindfulness practices incorporated into yoga, such as meditation and breath awareness, help women

cultivate mental clarity, emotional resilience, and a sense of calm amidst life's challenges.

3. **Improved Mood and Emotional Well-being:** Regular yoga practice is associated with enhanced mood and emotional well-being. The release of endorphins and other feel-good neurotransmitters during exercise, combined with the meditative aspects of yoga, uplifts spirits, promotes relaxation, and fosters a positive outlook on life.

4. **Enhanced Self-awareness:** Yoga encourages women to cultivate self-awareness by tuning into their bodies, thoughts, and emotions. Through mindful movement and introspection, women gain insight into their patterns of behavior, thought, and reaction, empowering them to make conscious choices that align with their values and intentions.

5. **Empowerment and Self-confidence:** As women progress in their yoga practice, they experience a sense of empowerment and self-confidence that extends beyond the mat. Mastering challenging poses, overcoming limitations, and embracing their unique strengths fosters a deep sense of self-belief and inner strength, empowering women to navigate life's obstacles with grace and resilience.

In essence, yoga offers women a holistic approach to physical and mental well-being, supporting them in leading healthier, happier lives. By incorporating yoga into their lifestyle, women can cultivate strength, flexibility, resilience, and inner peace, enhancing their overall quality of life and empowering them to thrive in all aspects of their journey.

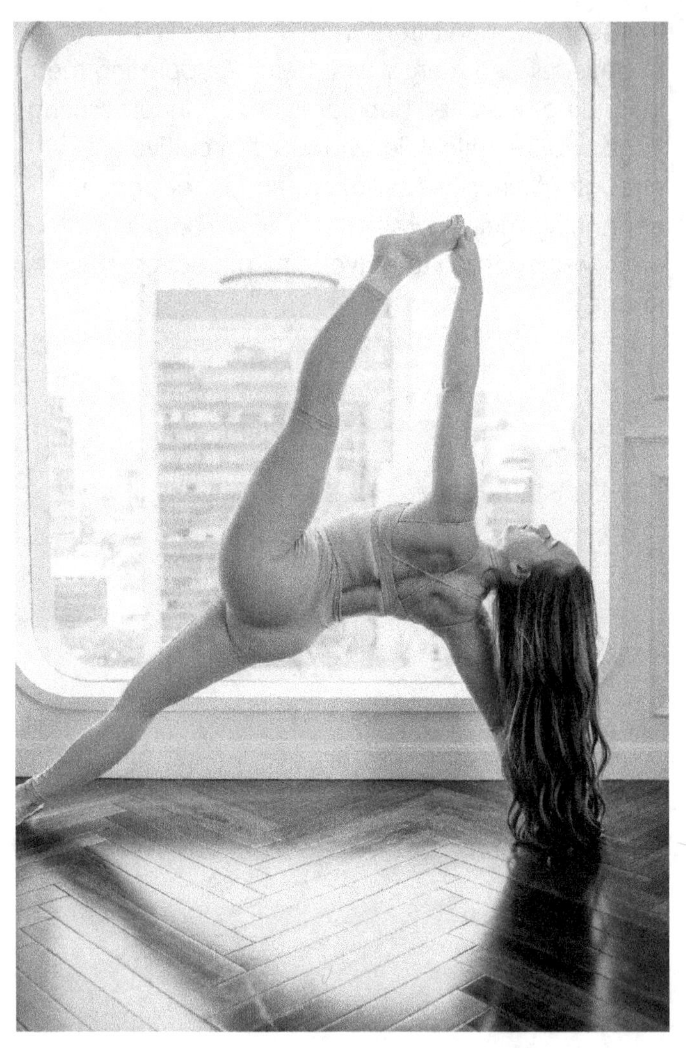

# CHAPTER ONE

## GETTING STARTED WITH YOGA

Getting started with yoga is an exciting journey that begins with a few key steps to ensure a comfortable and enjoyable experience. Here's a guide to help you embark on your yoga journey:

1. **Set Up Your Yoga Space:** Designate a quiet and clutter-free area in your home where you can practice yoga comfortably. Ideally, choose a space with ample natural light and enough room to move freely. Clear the area of any obstacles and create a calming atmosphere with soft lighting, candles, or soothing music if desired.

2. **Gather Your Yoga Equipment:** While yoga doesn't require a lot of equipment, having a few essentials can enhance your practice. Invest in a high-quality yoga mat that provides cushioning and grip to support your poses. You may also want to have yoga blocks, straps, and a bolster on hand to assist with alignment and deepen your stretches.

3. **Choose Comfortable Attire:** Wear lightweight and breathable clothing that allows for unrestricted movement. Opt for moisture-wicking fabrics that keep you cool and comfortable during your practice. Avoid overly loose or baggy clothing that may get in the way or restrict your movements.

4. **Start with Beginner-Friendly Resources:** If you're new to yoga, it's helpful to start with beginner-friendly resources to learn the basics. Consider attending a beginner's yoga class at a local studio or community center, where you can receive personalized instruction and guidance from a certified yoga instructor. Alternatively, explore online yoga platforms and mobile apps that offer beginner-level classes and tutorials.

5. **Learn Basic Yoga Poses:** Familiarize yourself with foundational yoga poses that form the building blocks of your practice. Start off by doing basic postures like Child's Pose (Balasana), Downward-Facing Dog (Adho Mukha Svanasana), and Mountain Pose (Tadasana). Focus on proper alignment, breathing, and mindful movement as you explore each pose.

6. **Practice Breathing Techniques:** Breath awareness is an integral aspect of yoga practice, helping to calm the mind, regulate emotions, and deepen relaxation. Learn basic breathing techniques such as diaphragmatic breathing (also known as belly breathing) and Ujjayi breath (ocean breath) to enhance your practice and cultivate mindfulness.

7. **Listen to Your Body:** As you begin your yoga practice, listen to your body and honor its needs. Avoid pushing yourself too hard or forcing

your body into uncomfortable positions. Instead, practice self-awareness and self-compassion, modifying poses as needed to suit your body's abilities and limitations.

8. **Be Patient and Persistent:** Yoga is a journey of self-discovery and continuous growth. Be patient with yourself as you progress in your practice, understanding that improvement takes time and consistency. Embrace the process with an open mind and a compassionate heart, celebrating each step forward along the way.

By following these steps and approaching your yoga practice with curiosity and dedication, you'll lay a solid foundation for a fulfilling and transformative journey of self-exploration and holistic well-being. Remember to approach your practice with joy, curiosity, and a sense of adventure, allowing yourself to experience the myriad benefits that yoga has to offer.

## SETTING UP YOUR YOGA SPACE

Setting up your yoga space is essential for creating a conducive environment that promotes relaxation, focus, and mindfulness during your practice. Here's how to set up your yoga space:

1. **Choose a Dedicated Area:** Select a quiet and clutter-free area in your home where you can

practice yoga without distractions. Ideally, choose a space with enough room to move freely and stretch out in all directions. It could be a spare room, a corner of your living room, or even a spot in your backyard if weather permits.

2. **Clear the Space:** Remove any clutter, furniture, or objects that may obstruct your movement or distract your focus. Clearing the space creates a sense of openness and tranquility, allowing you to fully immerse yourself in your practice.

3. **Create Ambiance:** Enhance the atmosphere of your yoga space by adding elements that promote relaxation and mindfulness. Consider incorporating soft lighting, such as lamps or candles, to create a warm and inviting glow. You can also bring in natural elements like plants or flowers to add freshness and vitality to the space.

4. **Set the Mood with Music:** Choose soothing music or nature sounds to create a calming backdrop for your practice. Ambient instrumental music, gentle chants, or nature sounds like ocean waves or bird songs can help quiet the mind and deepen your sense of relaxation.

5. **Use Props and Equipment:** Keep your yoga props and equipment nearby for easy access during your practice. This may include a yoga mat, blocks, straps, blankets, and bolsters. Arrange

them neatly in a designated area so you can easily reach for them as needed.

6. **Personalize Your Space:** Make your yoga space feel like your own personal sanctuary by adding meaningful touches that resonate with you. This could include inspiring quotes or affirmations, sacred objects, or images that evoke a sense of peace and serenity.

7. **Minimize Distractions:** Turn off electronic devices, mute notifications, and minimize external distractions to create a serene and focused environment. Let this time be a sacred space for you to disconnect from the outside world and reconnect with yourself.

8. **Create Rituals:** Establish rituals or routines that signal the beginning and end of your yoga practice. This could be lighting a candle, setting an intention, or practicing a few moments of mindfulness before and after your practice to transition mindfully into and out of your yoga space.

By setting up your yoga space thoughtfully and intentionally, you create a supportive environment that encourages relaxation, focus, and self-discovery during your practice. Take the time to cultivate a space that nourishes your body, mind, and spirit, and let it become a sanctuary where you can retreat to find peace and inner calm amidst the busyness of daily life.

# CHOOSING THE RIGHT YOGA MAT AND EQUIPMENT

Choosing the right yoga mat and equipment is essential for ensuring comfort, stability, and support during your yoga practice. Here's a guide to help you select the best yoga mat and accessories for your needs:

1. **Yoga Mat:**
   - **Thickness:** Yoga mats come in various thicknesses, typically ranging from 1/16 inch (1.5 mm) to 1/4 inch (6 mm). Thicker mats provide more cushioning for sensitive joints, while thinner mats offer better stability and connection to the ground.
   - **Material:** Consider the material of the yoga mat, as it affects grip, durability, and eco-friendliness. Common materials include PVC (polyvinyl chloride), TPE (thermoplastic elastomer), natural rubber, and cork. Choose a material that matches your choices and values.
   - **Texture:** Look for a yoga mat with a textured surface that provides grip and prevents slipping, especially when practicing challenging poses or in hot and sweaty conditions. Some mats feature a smooth surface, while others have a textured or sticky finish for added traction.
   - **Size:** Ensure that the yoga mat is long and wide enough to accommodate your body comfortably in various yoga poses. Standard yoga

mats typically measure around 68-72 inches (173-183 cm) in length and 24 inches (61 cm) in width, but you may opt for longer or wider mats if you prefer extra space.

2. **Yoga Props and Accessories:**
   - **Blocks:** Yoga blocks are used to provide support, stability, and extension in poses where flexibility or range of motion is limited. Choose blocks made from lightweight and durable materials like foam, cork, or bamboo.
   - **Straps:** Yoga straps assist in achieving proper alignment and deepening stretches by extending reach and providing support in poses that require flexibility. Look for adjustable straps made from soft, durable materials like cotton or nylon.
   - **Blankets:** Yoga blankets offer padding, warmth, and support during seated and reclining poses, as well as relaxation at the end of your practice. Opt for blankets made from natural fibers like cotton or wool for breathability and comfort.
   - **Bolsters:** Yoga bolsters are cylindrical cushions used to provide support and relaxation in restorative poses, meditation, and pranayama (breathing exercises). Choose bolsters with a firm yet plush feel and a removable, washable cover for easy maintenance.

3. **Consider Eco-Friendly Options:**
   - If sustainability is important to you, consider eco-friendly yoga mats and accessories made from

recycled materials, natural rubber, cork, or organic cotton. These options minimize environmental impact and align with your commitment to conscious consumption.

### 4. **Try Before You Buy:**
   - Whenever possible, test out different yoga mats and equipment in person to assess their comfort, grip, and suitability for your practice. Many yoga studios offer rental mats and props or provide samples for trial use during classes.

### 5. **Invest in Quality:**
   - While it may be tempting to opt for the cheapest option, investing in high-quality yoga mat and equipment ensures durability, performance, and longevity. Quality products offer better grip, support, and comfort, enhancing your overall yoga experience and preventing the need for frequent replacements.

By selecting the right yoga mat and equipment tailored to your preferences, needs, and values, you can create a supportive and comfortable environment that enhances your yoga practice and facilitates greater enjoyment, focus, and progress on the mat.

# SELECTING COMFORTABLE ATTIRE FOR YOGA PRACTICE

Selecting comfortable attire for your yoga practice is essential for ensuring freedom of movement, breathability, and ease during your practice. Here are some tips for choosing the right yoga attire:

1. **Moisture-Wicking Fabrics:** Opt for clothing made from moisture-wicking fabrics that draw sweat away from the skin and help keep you dry and comfortable during your practice. Look for materials like nylon, polyester, or spandex blends that offer stretch and breathability.

2. **Lightweight and Breathable:** Choose lightweight and breathable clothing that allows for unrestricted movement and ventilation. Avoid heavy or restrictive fabrics that may cause overheating or discomfort, especially during vigorous or heated yoga classes.

3. **Flexible and Stretchy:** Select clothing with a comfortable, stretchy fit that moves with your body and accommodates a wide range of motion. Look for leggings, shorts, or yoga pants with four-way stretch for maximum flexibility and freedom of movement.

4. **Form-Fitting but Not Restrictive:** While form-fitting clothing can help you maintain proper alignment and prevent distractions during your

practice, avoid garments that are overly tight or constrictive. Choose clothing that fits comfortably without restricting circulation or impeding movement.

5. **Layering Options:** Consider layering your yoga attire with breathable, moisture-wicking layers that you can easily remove or adjust as needed throughout your practice. This allows you to regulate your body temperature and stay comfortable during different phases of your practice, such as warm-up, active poses, and relaxation.

6. **Supportive Sports Bras:** For women, wearing a supportive sports bra is essential for comfort and confidence during yoga practice. Choose a sports bra that offers adequate support, coverage, and moisture-wicking properties to keep you feeling secure and comfortable throughout your practice.

7. **Minimalist Design:** Opt for clothing with a minimalist design and minimal seams or embellishments that may cause irritation or chafing during movement. Seamless or flat-lock seams help prevent friction and discomfort, especially in areas prone to rubbing or pressure points.

8. **Versatility for All Types of Yoga:** Select yoga attire that is versatile and suitable for various types of yoga practices, from gentle restorative

yoga to dynamic vinyasa flow or hot yoga. Choose clothing that offers comfort, support, and breathability across different styles and intensities of yoga.

9. **Personal Style and Expression:** Express your personal style and preferences through your choice of yoga attire, whether you prefer bold prints, vibrant colors, or understated neutrals. Wear clothing that makes you feel confident, empowered, and aligned with your intentions for your yoga practice.

10. **Comfortable Footwear:** In most yoga practices, practitioners typically practice barefoot or in grip socks to maintain stability and connection with the ground. However, if you prefer wearing footwear, choose lightweight and flexible shoes with minimal cushioning that allow for natural movement and proprioception.

By selecting comfortable, functional, and stylish attire tailored to your preferences and needs, you can enhance your yoga practice and create a supportive environment that allows you to move with ease, focus, and mindfulness on the mat.

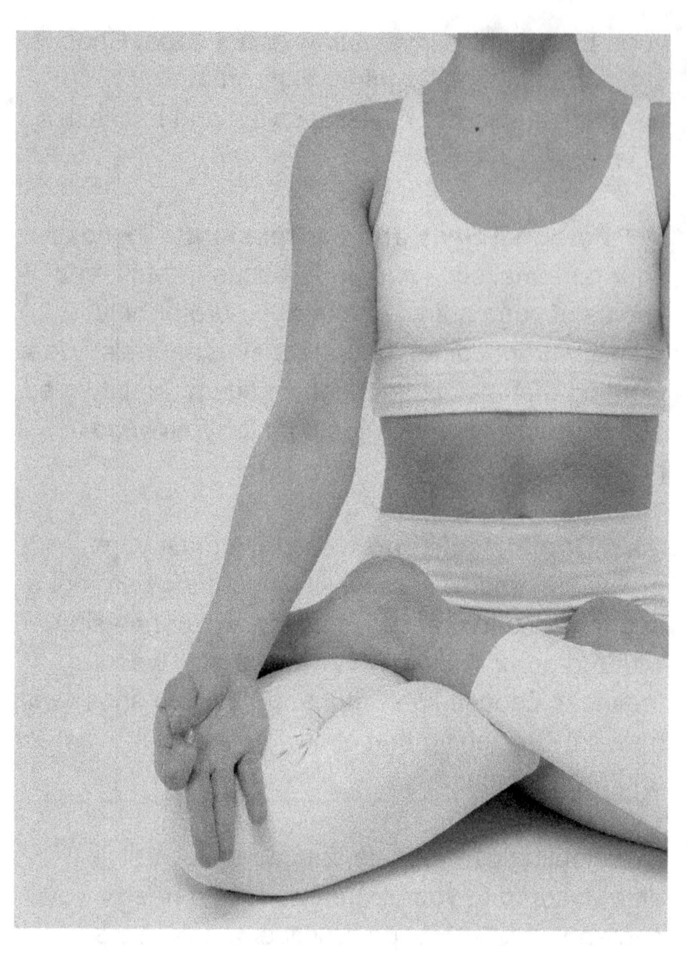

# CHAPTER TWO

## THE BASICS OF YOGA

The basics of yoga encompass fundamental principles, practices, and concepts that serve as the foundation for a holistic and transformative yoga journey. Here's an overview of the key components of the basics of yoga:

1. **Yoga Philosophy:** At the heart of yoga is a rich philosophical tradition that originated in ancient India. Central to yoga philosophy are foundational texts such as the Yoga Sutras of Patanjali, which outline the eight limbs of yoga (Ashtanga Yoga) as a path to spiritual liberation (Samadhi). These include ethical principles (Yamas and Niyamas), physical postures (Asanas), breath control (Pranayama), withdrawal of the senses (Pratyahara), concentration (Dharana), meditation (Dhyana), and ultimate absorption (Samadhi).

2. **Breath Awareness:** Breath awareness is a fundamental aspect of yoga practice, serving as a bridge between the body and the mind. Practicing conscious breathing techniques (Pranayama) helps regulate the breath, calm the mind, and cultivate present-moment awareness. Techniques such as deep belly breathing (Diaphragmatic Breath), Ujjayi Breath (Victorious Breath), and alternate nostril breathing (Nadi Shodhana) are commonly used in

yoga to enhance vitality, relaxation, and mental clarity.

3. **Yoga Asanas (Postures):** Yoga postures, or asanas, are physical poses that promote strength, flexibility, balance, and mindfulness. There is a wide variety of yoga asanas, ranging from standing poses, seated poses, forward bends, backbends, twists, inversions, and restorative poses. Each posture has specific physical and energetic benefits and can be modified or adapted to suit individual needs and abilities.

4. **Alignment and Safety:** Proper alignment is crucial in yoga to ensure safety, prevent injury, and maximize the benefits of each posture. Paying attention to alignment cues, such as engaging core muscles, maintaining a neutral spine, and aligning joints, helps practitioners practice yoga with integrity and awareness. Props such as yoga blocks, straps, and blankets can also be used to support alignment and enhance the effectiveness of yoga poses.

5. **Mindfulness and Meditation:** Yoga practice extends beyond the physical postures to include mindfulness and meditation practices that cultivate mental clarity, emotional balance, and inner peace. Mindfulness involves paying attention to the present moment with openness and acceptance, while meditation involves training the mind to focus and quiet the chatter of thoughts. Both practices

help reduce stress, enhance self-awareness, and deepen the connection between mind, body, and spirit.

6. **Relaxation and Savasana:** Every yoga practice typically concludes with a period of relaxation and integration known as Savasana (Corpse Pose). Savasana allows practitioners to rest deeply, release tension, and assimilate the benefits of their practice. It is a time for surrender, stillness, and inner reflection, providing an opportunity to experience deep relaxation and rejuvenation.

By embracing the basics of yoga—incorporating breath awareness, practicing yoga postures mindfully, and cultivating a sense of inner peace and well-being—practitioners can embark on a transformative journey of self-discovery, healing, and holistic wellness. Whether you're new to yoga or a seasoned practitioner, returning to the basics can deepen your practice and enrich your experience on and off the mat.

# UNDERSTANDING YOGA PHILOSOPHY AND PRINCIPLES

Understanding yoga philosophy and principles provides a deeper context for the practice, guiding practitioners on a path of self-discovery, personal growth, and spiritual evolution. Here's an overview of key elements of yoga philosophy and principles:

1. **The Eight Limbs of Yoga (Ashtanga Yoga):** Yoga philosophy is outlined in the Yoga Sutras of Patanjali, which describe the eight limbs of yoga as a systematic path to self-realization and liberation (Samadhi). The eight limbs are:
   - **Yamas:** Ethical guidelines for interacting with the world, including principles of non-violence (Ahimsa), truthfulness (Satya), non-stealing (Asteya), moderation (Brahmacharya), and non-possessiveness (Aparigraha).
   - **Niyamas:** Personal observances that cultivate self-discipline and inner purity, including practices of cleanliness (Shaucha), contentment (Santosha), self-discipline (Tapas), self-study (Svadhyaya), and surrender to a higher power (Ishvara Pranidhana).
   - **Asanas:** Physical postures that promote strength, flexibility, and balance in the body, preparing the practitioner for meditation and spiritual practices.
   - **Pranayama:** Breath control techniques that regulate the breath, calm the mind, and enhance vital energy (Prana).
   - **Pratyahara:** Withdrawal of the senses from external distractions, allowing the practitioner to turn inward and cultivate inner awareness.
   - **Dharana:** Concentration practices that focus the mind on a single point or object, developing mental discipline and concentration.

- **Dhyana:** Meditation practices that cultivate deep inner awareness, insight, and connection with the divine.
    - **Samadhi:** The ultimate state of spiritual absorption, where the practitioner experiences oneness with the divine and transcends the limitations of the ego.

2. **Karma Yoga, Bhakti Yoga, Jnana Yoga:** In addition to the eight limbs of yoga, there are various paths (Yogas) that cater to different temperaments and inclinations of practitioners:
    - **Karma Yoga:** The path of selfless action and service, where practitioners perform their duties without attachment to the fruits of their actions, dedicating their efforts to the greater good.
    - **Bhakti Yoga:** The path of devotion and love, where practitioners cultivate deep devotion and surrender to a higher power through prayer, worship, and acts of devotion.
    - **Jnana Yoga:** The path of knowledge and wisdom, where practitioners seek self-realization through self-inquiry, study of scriptures, and contemplation of philosophical truths.

3. **Yoga as Union:** At its core, yoga means union or integration—uniting the individual self (Atman) with the universal consciousness (Brahman). Yoga philosophy teaches that through the practices of yoga, practitioners can experience a sense of oneness and interconnectedness with all

of creation, transcending the illusion of separation and realizing their inherent divinity.

4. **Ahimsa and Non-Dualism:** Ahimsa, or non-violence, is a foundational principle of yoga philosophy, emphasizing compassion, kindness, and respect for all living beings. Yoga philosophy also teaches the principle of non-dualism (Advaita), which asserts that the true nature of reality is non-dual, beyond distinctions of good and bad, right and wrong, self and other.

By understanding and embodying the principles of yoga philosophy, practitioners can deepen their practice, cultivate greater self-awareness, and live with greater compassion, harmony, and integrity in their lives. Yoga becomes not just a physical practice but a way of living—a path to wholeness, fulfillment, and spiritual awakening.

## BREATHING TECHNIQUES (PRANAYAMA) FOR WOMEN

Pranayama, or yogic breathing techniques, offer numerous benefits for women's health and well-being, addressing both physical and emotional aspects of their experience. Here are several pranayama techniques that are particularly beneficial for women:

1. **Dirga Pranayama (Three-Part Breath):**
Dirga pranayama is a foundational breathing technique that encourages deep, diaphragmatic breathing. It involves breathing deeply into the abdomen, then expanding the ribcage, and finally filling the chest with air. This three-part breath helps women relax, reduce stress, and increase oxygenation throughout the body, promoting a sense of calm and centeredness.

2. **Nadi Shodhana (Alternate Nostril Breathing):** Nadi shodhana is a balancing and purifying pranayama technique that involves alternating the breath between the left and right nostrils. This practice helps balance the flow of energy (prana) in the body, harmonize the nervous system, and calm the mind. Nadi shodhana is particularly beneficial for women experiencing hormonal imbalances, menstrual irregularities, or mood swings.

3. **Bhramari Pranayama (Bee Breath):**
Bhramari pranayama is a soothing and grounding breathing technique that involves making a humming sound while exhaling. This practice helps quiet the mind, reduce anxiety, and promote relaxation. Bhramari pranayama can be especially helpful for women dealing with stress, insomnia, or emotional turmoil.

4. **Sitali Pranayama (Cooling Breath):** Sitali pranayama is a cooling and calming breathing

technique that involves inhaling through a rolled tongue or pursed lips, creating a cooling sensation in the mouth and throat. This practice helps regulate body temperature, reduce heat-related discomfort (such as hot flashes), and soothe inflammation or irritation in the throat.

**5. **Ujjayi Pranayama (Victorious Breath):****
Ujjayi pranayama is a rhythmic breathing technique that involves constricting the back of the throat slightly while inhaling and exhaling through the nose. This creates a gentle oceanic sound, which helps focus the mind, deepen concentration, and regulate the breath. Ujjayi pranayama can be particularly beneficial for women during labor and childbirth, helping them stay calm, centered, and connected to their breath.

**6. **Surya Bhedana and Chandra Bhedana:****
Surya bhedana (solar piercing breath) involves inhaling through the right nostril and exhaling through the left nostril, activating the sympathetic nervous system and increasing energy levels. Chandra bhedana (lunar piercing breath) involves inhaling through the left nostril and exhaling through the right nostril, activating the parasympathetic nervous system and promoting relaxation. Practicing these techniques in sequence can help women balance energy levels, regulate menstrual cycles, and support hormonal harmony.

**7. **Kapalabhati (Skull-Shining Breath):****
Kapalabhati is an invigorating pranayama
technique that involves rapid, forceful exhalations
followed by passive inhalations. This practice
increases circulation, stimulates digestion, and
energizes the body and mind. Kapalabhati can be
particularly beneficial for women experiencing
sluggishness, fatigue, or mental fog.

When practicing pranayama, it's essential for
women to listen to their bodies, start slowly, and
gradually increase the duration and intensity of their
practice over time. Pranayama can be incorporated
into a daily yoga routine or practiced on its own as
a standalone practice to promote balance, vitality,
and well-being for women of all ages and stages of
life.

# INTRODUCTION TO MEDITATION FOR WOMEN'S WELL-BEING

Meditation is a powerful practice that offers
numerous benefits for women's physical, mental,
and emotional well-being. Rooted in ancient
wisdom and supported by modern science,
meditation provides women with a practical tool to
cultivate inner peace, reduce stress, and enhance
overall quality of life. In this introduction to
meditation for women's well-being, we explore the
essence of meditation, its benefits, and how women

can integrate this practice into their lives to promote holistic wellness.

**Understanding Meditation:**
Meditation is a practice of focused attention and mindfulness that involves training the mind to cultivate a state of present-moment awareness and inner stillness. Through various meditation techniques, women can learn to observe their thoughts, emotions, and sensations without judgment, allowing them to cultivate greater clarity, balance, and resilience in the face of life's challenges.

**Benefits of Meditation for Women:**
Meditation offers a multitude of benefits tailored to women's unique needs and experiences. Some of the key benefits include:
- **Stress Reduction:** Meditation helps women manage stress more effectively by promoting relaxation, reducing cortisol levels, and calming the nervous system.
- **Emotional Balance:** Regular meditation practice enhances emotional resilience, reduces anxiety and depression symptoms, and fosters a greater sense of inner peace and contentment.
- **Improved Sleep:** Meditation can improve sleep quality and duration by promoting relaxation, reducing insomnia, and enhancing overall sleep hygiene.
- **Enhanced Mental Clarity:** Meditation sharpens mental focus, improves cognitive

function, and enhances concentration, helping women navigate daily tasks and challenges with greater clarity and efficiency.
- **Mind-Body Connection:** By deepening the connection between mind and body, meditation supports women's holistic wellness, promoting self-awareness, intuition, and self-care.

**Practical Tips for Starting a Meditation Practice:**
Getting started with meditation doesn't require any special equipment or prior experience. Here are some practical tips to help women begin their meditation journey:
- **Start Small:** Begin with short meditation sessions, such as 5-10 minutes, and gradually increase the duration as you become more comfortable with the practice.
- **Find a Quiet Space:** Choose a quiet and comfortable space where you can meditate without distractions. This could be a dedicated meditation corner in your home, a peaceful outdoor setting, or simply a quiet room with minimal noise.
- **Focus on the Breath:** Use the breath as a focal point for meditation, observing the natural rhythm of inhalation and exhalation. When the mind wanders, gently bring your attention back to the breath without judgment.
- **Explore Different Techniques:** Experiment with different meditation techniques, such as mindfulness meditation, loving-kindness meditation,

body scan meditation, or guided visualization, to find what resonates best with you.
- **Be Consistent:** Establish a regular meditation practice by setting aside time each day for meditation, whether it's first thing in the morning, during a lunch break, or before bedtime. Consistency is key to experiencing the full benefits of meditation over time.

**Conclusion:**
Meditation holds immense potential for women's well-being, offering a pathway to inner peace, resilience, and self-discovery. By integrating meditation into their daily lives, women can cultivate greater emotional balance, mental clarity, and overall vitality, empowering them to thrive in all aspects of their journey. As women embark on their meditation practice, they embark on a transformative journey of self-awareness, healing, and holistic wellness, unlocking the profound potential that lies within each moment of mindful presence.

# CHAPTER THREE

## ESSENTIAL YOGA POSES FOR WOMEN

Yoga offers a wide range of poses that cater to the specific needs and experiences of women, addressing physical health, mental well-being, and emotional balance. Here are ten essential yoga poses for women that promote strength, flexibility, relaxation, and overall vitality:

1. **Mountain Pose (Tadasana):** Mountain pose is a foundational standing pose that promotes alignment, balance, and grounding. Stand tall with your feet hip-width apart, arms by your sides, and palms facing forward. Mountain pose helps women cultivate stability, confidence, and a sense of inner strength.

2. **Forward Fold (Uttanasana):** Forward fold is a gentle forward bending pose that stretches the hamstrings, calves, and spine, while calming the mind and relieving stress. From mountain pose, hinge at the hips and fold forward, bringing your hands to the floor or resting them on your shins or thighs. Forward fold helps women release tension in the back and promote relaxation.

3. **Warrior II (Virabhadrasana II):** Warrior II is a dynamic standing pose that builds strength in the legs, opens the hips and chest, and cultivates mental focus and determination. From a wide-legged stance, turn one foot out to the side, bend the knee, and extend your arms out to the sides parallel to the floor. Warrior II empowers women to embrace their inner warrior and stand strong in their truth.

4. **Downward-Facing Dog (Adho Mukha Svanasana):** Downward-facing dog is a rejuvenating inversion that stretches the entire body, strengthens the arms and shoulders, and calms the mind. Start on your hands and knees, tuck your toes, and lift your hips toward the ceiling, forming an inverted V shape with your body. Downward dog helps women release tension in the back, shoulders, and hamstrings.

5. **Tree Pose (Vrksasana):** Tree pose is a balancing pose that strengthens the legs, improves focus and concentration, and promotes a sense of groundedness and stability. Stand tall on one foot, bring the sole of the other foot to rest on the inner thigh or calf, and bring your hands to your heart center or extend them overhead. Tree pose helps women cultivate balance, grace, and inner peace.

6. **Cobra Pose (Bhujangasana):** Cobra pose is a gentle backbend that strengthens the spine, opens the chest and heart center, and stimulates

the abdominal organs. Lie on your belly, place your hands under your shoulders, and lift your chest off the mat while keeping your elbows close to your body. Cobra pose helps women cultivate a sense of courage, vitality, and self-confidence.

7. **Seated Forward Bend (Paschimottanasana):** Seated forward bend is a calming pose that stretches the spine, hamstrings, and calves, while promoting introspection and surrender. Sit on the floor with your legs extended in front of you, hinge at the hips, and fold forward, reaching toward your feet. Seated forward bend helps women release tension in the body and mind, fostering relaxation and inner peace.

8. **Child's Pose (Balasana):** Child's pose is a resting pose that stretches the spine, hips, and shoulders, while calming the nervous system and promoting surrender and self-care. Kneel on the floor, sit back on your heels, and fold forward, resting your forehead on the mat and extending your arms overhead or by your sides. Child's pose offers women a sanctuary for rest, renewal, and introspection.

9. **Bridge Pose (Setu Bandhasana):** Bridge pose is a rejuvenating backbend that strengthens the back, glutes, and hamstrings, while opening the chest and heart center. Lie on your back with your knees bent and feet hip-width apart, lift your hips toward the ceiling, and clasp your hands under your

back. Bridge pose helps women cultivate strength, resilience, and a sense of expansiveness.

**10. **Corpse Pose (Savasana):**** Corpse pose is a final relaxation pose that allows the body and mind to integrate the benefits of the practice, promoting deep relaxation, surrender, and inner peace. Lie on your back with your arms and legs extended, palms facing up, and close your eyes. Surrender fully to the present moment, allowing tension to melt away and experiencing a sense of serenity and wholeness.

These essential yoga poses offer women a holistic approach to health and well-being, addressing physical strength, mental clarity, and emotional balance. Incorporate these poses into your yoga practice to cultivate vitality, resilience, and a deeper connection to yourself and the world around you.

## STANDING POSE FOR BALANCE AND STABILITY

A standing pose that enhances balance and stability is crucial for women's overall well-being, promoting physical strength and mental focus. One such pose is Tree Pose (Vrksasana). Here's how to practice it:

**1. **Start in Mountain Pose:**** Begin by standing tall with your feet hip-width apart, arms by your sides, and your gaze forward. Feel the connection of your feet with the ground, rooting down through all four corners of each foot.

2. **Shift Your Weight:** Shift your weight onto your left foot and bring your right foot to rest on the inside of your left thigh. You can place the sole of your right foot against your inner left thigh, calf, or ankle—avoid placing it directly on the knee joint to prevent strain.

3. **Find Your Balance:** Engage your core muscles to stabilize your pelvis and lengthen through your spine. Press your left foot firmly into the ground and actively lift through your chest. Find a focal point—a drishti—either in front of you or on the floor, to help maintain your balance and focus.

4. **Choose Your Arms Position:** Bring your hands together in front of your heart center in prayer position (Anjali Mudra), or extend your arms overhead with your palms facing each other, reaching toward the sky like the branches of a tree.

5. **Hold and Breathe:** Hold the pose for several breaths, finding a steady gaze and maintaining a soft, steady breath. Feel the stability and strength of your standing leg, and the groundedness of your foot pressing into the earth.

6. **Release and Repeat:** Release the pose gently, returning your right foot to the ground, and then switch sides, placing your right foot firmly on

the ground and bringing your left foot to rest on the inside of your right thigh. Repeat the pose on the other side.

Tree Pose strengthens the muscles of the standing leg, improves balance and coordination, and cultivates a sense of inner stability and rootedness. Practice this pose regularly to enhance your balance and stability, both on and off the yoga mat.

# SEATED POSES FOR FLEXIBILITY AND RELAXATION

Seated poses are excellent for promoting flexibility, relaxation, and inner calm, making them perfect for women looking to unwind and release tension from both body and mind. Here are some seated yoga poses that focus on flexibility and relaxation:

1. **Seated Forward Bend (Paschimottanasana):** Sit on the floor with your legs extended in front of you. Inhale to lengthen your spine, then exhale to hinge forward from the hips, reaching for your feet or shins. Keep your back straight and chest open as you fold forward, relaxing your neck and shoulders. This pose stretches the spine, hamstrings, and calves, promoting relaxation and introspection.

2. **Bound Angle Pose (Baddha Konasana):** Sit on the floor with the soles of your feet together

and knees bent out to the sides. Hold your feet or ankles with your hands, lengthen your spine, and gently press your knees toward the ground. Allow your hips to open and relax into the pose, feeling a gentle stretch in the inner thighs and groin. Bound angle pose releases tension in the hips and lower back, promoting relaxation and flexibility.

3. **Seated Twist (Ardha Matsyendrasana):** Sit on the floor with your legs extended in front of you. Bend your right knee and place your right foot on the outside of your left thigh. Inhale to lengthen your spine, then exhale to twist to the right, placing your left elbow on the outside of your right knee and reaching your right hand behind you. Hold the twist for a few breaths before repeating on the opposite side. Seated twist stretches the spine, shoulders, and hips, while promoting relaxation and detoxification.

4. **Seated Wide-Legged Forward Bend (Upavistha Konasana):** Sit on the floor with your legs extended wide apart. Inhale to lengthen your spine, then exhale to hinge forward from the hips, reaching for your feet or shins. Keep your back straight and chest open as you fold forward, relaxing your neck and shoulders. Seated wide-legged forward bend stretches the inner thighs, hamstrings, and spine, promoting relaxation and openness.

5. **Half Lord of the Fishes Pose (Ardha Matsyendrasana):** Sit on the floor with your legs extended in front of you. Bend your right knee and place your right foot on the outside of your left thigh. Inhale to lengthen your spine, then exhale to twist to the right, placing your left elbow on the outside of your right knee and reaching your right hand behind you. Hold the twist for a few breaths before repeating on the opposite side. Half Lord of the Fishes Pose stretches the spine, shoulders, and hips, while promoting relaxation and detoxification.

6. **Easy Pose (Sukhasana):** Sit on the floor with your legs crossed and your hands resting on your knees. Close your eyes and focus on your breath, allowing your body to relax and soften with each exhale. Easy pose is a simple seated posture that promotes relaxation, mindfulness, and inner calm.

Incorporate these seated yoga poses into your practice to improve flexibility, release tension, and cultivate a sense of relaxation and well-being. Practice with awareness and listen to your body's cues, moving gently and mindfully into each pose.

# SUPINE AND PRONE POSES FOR STRENGTH AND ALIGNMENT

Supine and prone poses, which involve lying on the back (supine) or on the front (prone), are excellent for building strength, improving alignment, and enhancing overall body awareness. Here are some supine and prone yoga poses that focus on strength and alignment:

**Supine Poses:**

1. **Bridge Pose (Setu Bandhasana):** Lie on your back with your knees bent and feet hip-width apart. Press into your feet to lift your hips toward the ceiling, engaging your glutes and thighs. You can clasp your hands under your back for support or keep them by your sides. Bridge pose strengthens the back, glutes, and hamstrings, while improving spinal flexibility and alignment.

2. **Supine Twist (Supta Matsyendrasana):** Lie on your back with your knees bent and feet flat on the floor. Extend your arms out to the sides in a T position. Exhale to lower both knees to one side, keeping your shoulders grounded. Hold the twist for a few breaths, then switch sides. Supine twist stretches the spine, shoulders, and chest, while promoting spinal alignment and detoxification.

3. **Corpse Pose (Savasana):** Lie on your back with your legs extended and arms by your sides,

palms facing up. Close your eyes and allow your body to relax completely, releasing tension in every muscle. Corpse pose promotes deep relaxation, stress relief, and alignment of the spine.

**Prone Poses:**

1. **Cobra Pose (Bhujangasana):** Lie on your stomach with your palms flat on the mat under your shoulders. Inhale to lift your chest off the mat, keeping your elbows close to your body. Press the tops of your feet into the mat and use your leg muscles. Cobra pose strengthens the back, shoulders, and arms, while improving spinal flexibility and alignment.

2. **Locust Pose (Salabhasana):** Lie on your stomach with your arms by your sides and forehead resting on the mat. Inhale to lift your chest, arms, and legs off the mat, reaching back through your toes and fingers. Keep your gaze down to avoid straining the neck. Locust pose strengthens the back muscles, glutes, and hamstrings, while improving posture and spinal alignment.

3. **Bow Pose (Dhanurasana):** Lie on your stomach with your arms by your sides. Bend your knees and reach your hands back to grasp your ankles. Inhale to lift your chest and thighs off the mat, kicking your feet into your hands to deepen the stretch. Bow pose strengthens the back

muscles, opens the chest, and improves spinal
flexibility and alignment.

Incorporate these supine and prone yoga poses
into your practice to build strength, improve
alignment, and enhance overall body awareness.
Practice with mindfulness and listen to your body's
cues, moving gently and with intention into each
pose.

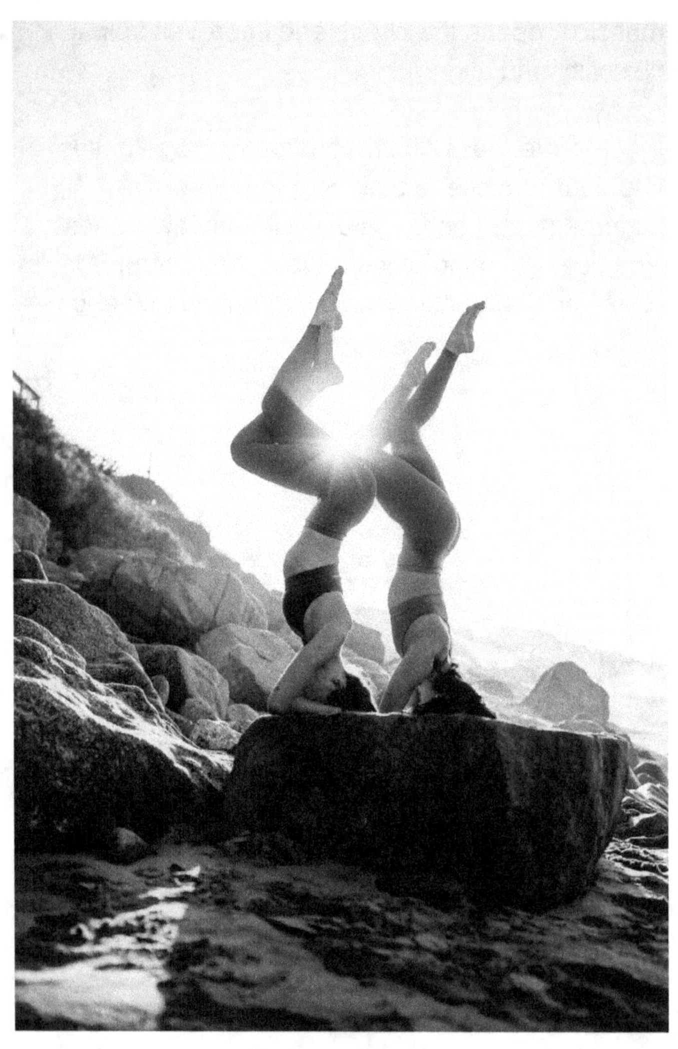

# CHAPTER FOUR

## INTERMEDIATE YOGA PRACTICES

Intermediate yoga practices build upon the foundation established in beginner-level classes, offering a more challenging and dynamic sequence of poses to deepen your practice. Here's an intermediate yoga sequence that focuses on strength, flexibility, balance, and mindfulness:

1. **Sun Salutations (Surya Namaskar):** Begin standing at the top of your mat. Inhale, raise your arms overhead, and arch back slightly (Mountain Pose). Exhale, fold forward into Uttanasana (Forward Fold). Inhale and lift halfway up with a flat back. Exhale, step or jump back to Chaturanga Dandasana (Low Plank). Inhale, lift into Upward-Facing Dog. Exhale, press back into Downward-Facing Dog. Repeat for several rounds, flowing with your breath.

2. **Warrior I (Virabhadrasana I):** From Downward-Facing Dog, step your right foot forward between your hands. Spin your back foot flat at a 45-degree angle. Inhale, reach your arms overhead, stacking your shoulders over your hips. Square your hips forward and gaze up. Hold for a few breaths before repeating on the opposite side.

3. **Warrior II (Virabhadrasana II):** From Warrior I, open your hips and arms to the side, extending your arms parallel to the floor. Stack your front knee over your ankle while keeping it bent. Gaze over your front fingertips. Hold for a few breaths before repeating on the opposite side.

4. **Triangle Pose (Trikonasana):** From Warrior II, straighten your front leg and reach your front arm forward, lowering it to rest on your shin, ankle, or the floor. Extend your top arm toward the sky, stacking your shoulders. Keep your chest open and gaze up or down. Hold for a few breaths before repeating on the opposite side.

5. **Pigeon Pose (Eka Pada Rajakapotasana):** From Downward-Facing Dog, bring your right knee forward and place it behind your right wrist, extending your left leg back. Square your hips and fold forwards over your front leg. Hold for a few breaths before repeating on the opposite side.

6. **Boat Pose (Navasana):** Sit on the mat with your knees bent and feet flat on the floor. Lean back slightly, engage your core, and lift your feet off the mat, bringing your shins parallel to the floor. Extend your arms forwards beside your legs, palms facing each other. Hold for several breaths, then release.

7. **Camel Pose (Ustrasana):** Kneel on the mat with your knees hip-width apart. With your fingers pointed down, place your hands on your lower back. Inhale, lift your chest, and arch back, reaching your hands toward your heels. Keep your hips stacked over your knees and gaze up. Hold for several breaths, then release.

8. **Shoulder Stand (Sarvangasana):** Lie on your back with your arms by your sides, palms facing down. Lift your legs toward the ceiling, then press your hands into the mat and lift your hips off the ground, coming into Shoulder Stand. Keep your gaze toward your toes and hold for several breaths. Slowly lower down with control.

9. **Corpse Pose (Savasana):** Lie on your back with your legs extended and arms by your sides, palms facing up. Close your eyes and allow your body to fully relax, sinking into the mat. Stay here for several minutes, focusing on your breath and letting go of tension.

This intermediate yoga sequence combines dynamic movement with mindful awareness, offering a balanced practice that challenges both the body and the mind. Practice at your own pace, listening to your body and honoring its needs as you explore each pose.

# DEEPENING YOUR PRACTICE WITH INTERMEDIATE POSES

Deepening your yoga practice involves exploring more challenging poses that require increased strength, flexibility, and concentration. Intermediate poses offer an opportunity to expand your practice and cultivate a deeper connection between mind, body, and breath. Here are some intermediate yoga poses to help you deepen your practice:

1. **Extended Side Angle Pose (Utthita Parsvakonasana):** From Warrior II, lower your front forearm to your thigh or reach your hand to the outside of your front foot. Extend your top arm overhead, creating a straight line from your back foot to your fingertips. This pose helps to strengthen the legs, open the hips, and extend the side body.

2. **Revolved Triangle Pose (Parivrtta Trikonasana):** From Triangle Pose, place your bottom hand on the outside of your front foot and reach your top arm toward the ceiling, twisting your torso open. Keep both legs straight and engage your core to maintain stability. Revolved Triangle strengthens the legs, improves spinal mobility, and aids in detoxification.

3. **Half Moon Pose (Ardha Chandrasana):** From Warrior II, shift your weight onto your front leg and bring your back foot off the mat, extending it

parallel to the floor. Place your bottom hand on the mat or a block under your shoulder, and extend your top arm toward the ceiling, creating a straight line from your back heel to your fingertips. Half Moon Pose improves balance, strengthens the legs and core, and opens the chest and shoulders.

4. **Crow Pose (Bakasana):** Start in a squatting position with your feet hip-width apart. Place your hands on the mat shoulder-width apart, spread your fingers wide, and lean forward, shifting your weight onto your hands. Lift your hips and bend your elbows, bringing your knees to rest on the backs of your upper arms. Engage your core and gaze forward. Crow Pose builds arm and core strength, improves balance, and cultivates focus and concentration.

5. **Wheel Pose (Urdhva Dhanurasana):** Lie on your back with your knees bent and feet hip-width apart, heels close to your hips. Place your hands by your ears with fingers pointing toward your shoulders. Press into your hands and feet to lift your hips toward the ceiling, coming into a backbend. Keep your arms and legs strong and engage your glutes and thighs. Wheel Pose strengthens the back, shoulders, and arms, improves spinal flexibility, and energizes the body.

6. **Forearm Stand (Pincha Mayurasana):** Start in Dolphin Pose with your forearms on the mat and your palms pressing into the floor. Walk your feet in

toward your elbows, stacking your hips over your shoulders. Lift one leg toward the ceiling, then the other, coming into Forearm Stand. Keep your core engaged and gaze between your forearms. Forearm Stand builds upper body and core strength, improves balance, and boosts confidence.

7. **Firefly Pose (Tittibhasana):** Begin in a squatting position with your feet slightly wider than hip-width apart. Place your hands on the floor between your feet and lean forward, lifting your hips and extending your legs toward the ceiling. Bring your knees to rest on the backs of your upper arms and engage your core. Firefly Pose strengthens the arms, core, and inner thighs, improves balance, and cultivates mental focus.

8. **Flying Pigeon Pose (Eka Pada Galavasana):** Start in Downward-Facing Dog and lift one leg toward the ceiling. Bend your lifted knee and draw it toward your chest, then lean forward and shift your weight into your hands, hooking your foot behind your upper arm. Extend your bottom leg back and engage your core. Flying Pigeon Pose strengthens the arms, core, and hip flexors, improves balance, and opens the hips.

As you explore these intermediate yoga poses, remember to approach them with patience, mindfulness, and self-compassion. Listen to your body, honor its limitations, and respect its boundaries. With consistent practice and dedication, you can deepen your yoga practice and experience the transformative benefits of these challenging poses.

## EXPLORING INVERSION AND ARM BALANCES SAFELY

Exploring inversions and arm balances can be exhilarating and empowering, but it's essential to approach these poses with caution and mindfulness to prevent injury. Here are some tips for safely exploring inversions and arm balances in your yoga practice:

1. **Build Core Strength:** Strong core muscles are essential for maintaining stability and control in inversions and arm balances. Incorporate core-strengthening exercises such as plank pose, boat pose, and forearm plank into your regular practice to build strength and stability.

2. **Warm-Up Properly:** Always warm up your body before attempting inversions and arm balances. Start with gentle stretches and movements to prepare your muscles and joints, focusing particularly on the wrists, shoulders, and core.

3. **Use Props:** Props such as blocks, straps, and bolsters can provide support and stability as you explore inversions and arm balances. Use

props to modify poses and gradually work towards more advanced variations.

**4. **Practice Against a Wall:**** Practicing inversions and arm balances against a wall can provide support and prevent falls. Start by practicing poses like handstand and forearm stand with your back to the wall, gradually working towards balancing away from the wall as you gain confidence and strength.

**5. **Engage Your Core:**** Strong engagement of the core muscles is key to maintaining stability and control in inversions and arm balances. Focus on drawing your navel towards your spine and lifting your pelvic floor to create a strong foundation of support.

**6. **Mind Your Alignment:**** Pay close attention to your alignment in inversions and arm balances to avoid putting unnecessary strain on your joints. Keep your wrists, elbows, and shoulders stacked and aligned, and avoid collapsing into the shoulders or rounding the spine.

**7. **Practice Mindful Breathing:**** Maintain a steady and controlled breath while practicing inversions and arm balances. Deep, steady breaths can help calm the mind, focus your attention, and provide a sense of stability and ease in challenging poses.

**8. **Listen to Your Body:**** Pay attention to how your body feels in inversions and arm balances, and honor any sensations of discomfort or strain. If a pose feels too challenging or causes pain, back off and explore a gentler variation or modify the pose with props.

**9. **Work with a Qualified Teacher:**** If you're new to inversions and arm balances, consider working with a qualified yoga teacher who can provide personalized guidance, alignment cues, and hands-on assistance to help you explore these poses safely and effectively.

**10. **Practice Patience and Persistence:****
Learning inversions and arm balances takes time, patience, and consistent practice. Approach your practice with curiosity, humility, and a willingness to explore and grow at your own pace.

By following these tips and practicing with mindfulness and awareness, you can safely explore inversions and arm balances, expand your practice, and experience the transformative benefits of these empowering poses. Remember to always prioritize safety and listen to your body's wisdom as you journey into new and challenging territory in your yoga practice.

# ENHANCING FLEXIBILITY AND STRENGTH WITH FLOW SEQUENCES

Flow sequences are dynamic and fluid sequences of yoga poses that are linked together with the breath, creating a moving meditation that enhances flexibility, strength, and overall well-being. Here's how to create a flow sequence that focuses on enhancing flexibility and strength:

1. **Warm-Up:** Start your flow sequence with a gentle warm-up to prepare your body for movement. Begin in a comfortable seated position, close your eyes, and take several deep breaths, focusing on calming the mind and connecting with your breath. Then, move through gentle stretches and movements to warm up the spine, shoulders, hips, and legs.

2. **Sun Salutations (Surya Namaskar):** Sun salutations are a classic sequence of poses that link movement with breath, warming up the entire body and building strength and flexibility. Flow through several rounds of sun salutations, moving smoothly from one pose to the next with each inhale and exhale.

3. **Standing Poses:** Incorporate a variety of standing poses to build strength, stability, and flexibility in the legs, hips, and core. Include poses such as Warrior I, Warrior II, Extended Side Angle

Pose, Triangle Pose, and Tree Pose. Flow mindfully from one standing pose to the next, focusing on smooth transitions and steady breath.

4. **Balancing Poses:** Balancing poses challenge your stability and focus, enhancing both physical and mental strength. Include balancing poses such as Tree Pose, Eagle Pose, Half Moon Pose, and Warrior III. Focus on engaging your core and finding a steady gaze to help you maintain balance and stability.

5. **Backbends:** Backbends open the chest, stretch the front of the body, and build strength in the back muscles. Include poses such as Cobra Pose, Upward-Facing Dog, Camel Pose, and Bridge Pose. Move mindfully into each backbend, focusing on lengthening the spine and opening the heart.

6. **Forward Folds:** Forward folds stretch the hamstrings, calves, and lower back, promoting flexibility and relaxation. Include poses such as Forward Fold, Seated Forward Bend, Wide-Legged Forward Fold, and Standing Forward Bend. Allow your breath to guide you deeper into each forward fold, surrendering tension with each exhale.

7. **Twists:** Twisting poses wring out tension from the spine, improve digestion, and detoxify the body. Include poses such as Seated Twist, Revolved Triangle Pose, Revolved Side Angle

Pose, and Twisted Chair Pose. Move into each twist with awareness, lengthening the spine on the inhale and deepening the twist on the exhale.

8. **Cool Down:** Finish your flow sequence with a gentle cool down to help your body relax and restore after the dynamic movement. Include gentle stretches for the spine, hips, and shoulders, as well as relaxation poses such as Child's Pose, Supine Twist, and Corpse Pose.

9. **Final Relaxation:** End your flow sequence with a few moments of final relaxation in Corpse Pose (Savasana), allowing your body to rest and integrate the benefits of your practice. Close your eyes, release any tension in the body, and let go of any thoughts or distractions, allowing yourself to fully surrender and be present in the moment.

By incorporating these elements into your flow sequence and practicing with mindfulness and awareness, you can enhance both flexibility and strength, leaving you feeling energized, balanced, and revitalized. Experiment with different poses and sequences to find what works best for your body and needs, and remember to listen to your body's wisdom as you explore and grow in your practice.

# CHAPTER FIVE

## YOGA FOR WOMEN'S HEALTH AND WELLNESS

Yoga offers numerous benefits for women's health and wellness, addressing physical, mental, and emotional well-being. Here's how yoga can support women's health:

1. **Menstrual Health:** Certain yoga poses can help alleviate menstrual discomfort and promote hormonal balance. Poses such as Child's Pose, Supine Twist, and Reclining Bound Angle Pose can help relieve cramps, while gentle, restorative poses can provide comfort and relaxation during menstruation.

2. **Fertility:** Yoga can support fertility by reducing stress, balancing hormones, and improving blood flow to the reproductive organs. Practices that focus on opening the hips, such as Pigeon Pose and Butterfly Pose, can be particularly beneficial for women trying to conceive.

3. **Prenatal Yoga:** Prenatal yoga is specifically designed to support women during pregnancy, helping to alleviate common discomforts such as back pain, swelling, and fatigue. Prenatal yoga practices focus on gentle stretches, strengthening

poses, and breathing techniques to prepare the body and mind for childbirth.

4. **Postnatal Recovery:** Yoga can aid in postnatal recovery by strengthening the pelvic floor, improving core strength, and relieving tension in the body. Postnatal yoga practices focus on gentle movements, pelvic floor exercises, and breathwork to support the body as it heals and adjusts to motherhood.

5. **Bone Health:** Weight-bearing yoga poses can help improve bone density and reduce the risk of osteoporosis in women. Poses such as Warrior II, Triangle Pose, and Chair Pose can help strengthen the bones and muscles, promoting overall bone health.

6. **Heart Health:** Yoga can benefit cardiovascular health by reducing stress, lowering blood pressure, and improving circulation. Practices that incorporate dynamic movements, such as Sun Salutations, can help improve cardiovascular fitness and support heart health.

7. **Stress Reduction:** Yoga is well-known for its ability to reduce stress and promote relaxation. Mindfulness practices, such as meditation and deep breathing techniques, can help women manage stress, anxiety, and overwhelm, fostering a sense of calm and well-being.

**8. **Emotional Balance:**** Yoga can support emotional balance by helping women connect with their inner selves, cultivate self-awareness, and develop coping strategies for managing emotions. Practices that focus on heart-opening poses, such as Camel Pose and Fish Pose, can help release tension and promote emotional healing.

**9. **Self-Care:**** Yoga encourages women to prioritize self-care and make time for themselves amidst their busy lives. Setting aside dedicated time for yoga practice allows women to nurture their physical, mental, and emotional well-being, promoting a greater sense of balance and fulfillment.

**10. **Community and Support:**** Yoga communities provide women with a supportive and nurturing environment where they can connect with like-minded individuals, share experiences, and receive encouragement and guidance on their wellness journey.

Overall, yoga offers women a holistic approach to health and wellness, supporting them through every stage of life with practices that nurture the body, calm the mind, and uplift the spirit. By incorporating yoga into their lives, women can cultivate greater vitality, resilience, and joy, allowing them to thrive in all aspects of their lives.

# YOGA FOR MENSTRUAL HEALTH AND HORMONAL BALANCE

Yoga can be a valuable tool for promoting menstrual health and hormonal balance in women. By incorporating specific poses, breathing techniques, and mindfulness practices into your routine, you can support your body's natural rhythms and alleviate discomfort associated with menstruation. Here are some ways yoga can help:

1. **Gentle Movement:** Gentle, restorative yoga poses can help alleviate menstrual cramps and discomfort by increasing blood flow to the pelvic region and releasing tension in the muscles. Poses such as Child's Pose, Supine Twist, and Cat-Cow Pose are particularly beneficial during menstruation.

2. **Hip-Opening Poses:** Hip-opening poses can help relieve tension in the hips and lower back, where many women experience discomfort during menstruation. Poses such as Pigeon Pose, Butterfly Pose, and Happy Baby Pose can help stretch and release tight muscles, promoting relaxation and comfort.

3. **Forward Folds:** Forward folding poses can help calm the nervous system and promote relaxation, which can be beneficial for managing menstrual symptoms such as anxiety and irritability. Poses such as Seated Forward Bend, Standing

Forward Bend, and Wide-Legged Forward Fold can help soothe the mind and body during menstruation.

4. **Breathing Techniques:** Pranayama, or yogic breathing techniques, can help regulate the nervous system and promote a sense of calm and balance. Deep, diaphragmatic breathing can help alleviate stress and tension, while alternate nostril breathing (Nadi Shodhana) can help balance hormones and calm the mind.

5. **Restorative Yoga:** Restorative yoga poses involve gentle, supported stretches that allow the body to relax deeply and release tension. Practicing restorative yoga poses such as Legs-Up-the-Wall Pose, Supported Bridge Pose, and Supported Reclining Bound Angle Pose can help promote relaxation and ease discomfort during menstruation.

6. **Mindfulness and Meditation:** Mindfulness practices such as meditation and guided visualization can help women connect with their bodies and cultivate a sense of acceptance and ease during menstruation. Taking time to sit quietly, breathe deeply, and observe sensations in the body can help promote hormonal balance and emotional well-being.

7. **Regular Practice:** Consistent yoga practice, especially during the menstrual cycle, can help

regulate hormones, reduce stress, and support overall menstrual health. By incorporating yoga into your routine on a regular basis, you can create a sense of balance and harmony in your body and mind.

It's important to listen to your body and honor its needs during menstruation. If you're experiencing severe pain or discomfort, it's essential to consult with a healthcare provider to rule out any underlying medical conditions. With regular yoga practice and mindful self-care, you can support your menstrual health and promote hormonal balance naturally.

# PRENATAL AND POSTNATAL FOR EXPECTING AND NEW MOTHERS

Prenatal and postnatal yoga offer valuable support and benefits for expecting and new mothers, helping to promote physical comfort, emotional well-being, and connection with the baby. Here's how prenatal and postnatal yoga can benefit expecting and new mothers:

**Prenatal Yoga:**

1. **Physical Comfort:** Prenatal yoga focuses on gentle stretches and movements that help alleviate common discomforts of pregnancy such as back pain, hip tightness, and swelling. Poses are

modified to accommodate the changing needs and limitations of the pregnant body.

2. **Stress Reduction:** Pregnancy can bring about significant physical and emotional changes, and prenatal yoga provides a safe space for mothers to relax, breathe, and connect with their baby. Mindfulness practices and breathing techniques help reduce stress and anxiety, promoting a sense of calm and well-being.

3. **Preparation for Childbirth:** Prenatal yoga teaches mothers valuable tools and techniques to prepare for childbirth, including breathing techniques, pelvic floor exercises, and positions for labor and delivery. These practices can help increase confidence and reduce fear surrounding childbirth.

4. **Connection with Baby:** Prenatal yoga provides an opportunity for mothers to deepen their connection with their baby through mindfulness practices and gentle movements. Poses such as Cat-Cow Pose and Pigeon Pose can help mothers tune into their body and connect with the life growing within them.

5. **Community Support:** Prenatal yoga classes often provide a supportive community of other expecting mothers, creating a space for sharing experiences, offering support, and building

friendships with others going through a similar journey.

**Postnatal Yoga:**

1. **Physical Recovery:** Postnatal yoga focuses on supporting the body's recovery after childbirth, helping to strengthen the core, pelvic floor, and other muscles that may have been weakened during pregnancy and childbirth. Gentle stretches and movements help relieve tension and promote healing.

2. **Emotional Support:** The postpartum period can be challenging emotionally, and postnatal yoga offers a safe and nurturing space for mothers to process their feelings, release stress, and cultivate self-compassion. Mindfulness practices and relaxation techniques help mothers navigate the emotional ups and downs of new motherhood.

3. **Bonding with Baby:** Postnatal yoga classes often incorporate poses and movements that involve the baby, providing an opportunity for mothers to bond with their baby while practicing yoga. Baby-friendly poses such as Baby Cobra Pose and Baby Boat Pose allow mothers to engage with their baby in a playful and nurturing way.

4. **Self-Care:** Taking time for self-care is essential for new mothers, and postnatal yoga provides an opportunity for mothers to prioritize

their own well-being amidst the demands of caring for a newborn. Practicing yoga allows mothers to recharge, replenish, and reconnect with themselves.

5. **Community Connection:** Postnatal yoga classes offer a supportive community of other new mothers, providing a space for sharing experiences, offering encouragement, and building friendships. Connecting with other mothers who are going through similar experiences can be incredibly validating and empowering.

Overall, prenatal and postnatal yoga offer valuable support and benefits for expecting and new mothers, helping them navigate the physical, emotional, and spiritual journey of pregnancy, childbirth, and new motherhood with greater ease, grace, and resilience.

# YOGA FOR WOMEN'S MENTAL HEALTH AND EMOTIONAL WELL-BEING

Yoga can be a powerful tool for supporting women's mental health and emotional well-being, providing a holistic approach to self-care and healing. Here's how yoga can benefit women's mental health and emotional well-being:

1. **Stress Reduction:** Yoga helps reduce stress by activating the body's relaxation response through mindful movement, deep breathing, and relaxation techniques. Practices such as gentle yoga, restorative yoga, and yoga nidra promote relaxation, soothe the nervous system, and calm the mind.

2. **Anxiety Management:** Yoga offers effective tools for managing anxiety by promoting mindfulness, grounding, and presence in the moment. Breathing techniques such as diaphragmatic breathing, alternate nostril breathing, and deep belly breathing can help regulate the nervous system and reduce feelings of anxiety.

3. **Depression Relief:** Yoga can help alleviate symptoms of depression by increasing levels of feel-good neurotransmitters such as serotonin and dopamine, improving mood, and promoting a sense of well-being. Practices such as heart-opening poses, backbends, and inversions can help lift the spirits and cultivate a positive outlook.

4. **Emotional Regulation:** Yoga teaches women how to navigate and regulate their emotions by cultivating self-awareness, self-compassion, and acceptance of their inner experience. Mindfulness practices such as meditation, body scans, and mindful movement help women develop a deeper connection with themselves and their emotions.

5. **Self-Compassion:** Yoga encourages women to practice self-compassion and kindness towards themselves, fostering a sense of self-love and acceptance. Through yoga, women learn to treat themselves with gentleness, patience, and understanding, even in times of difficulty or struggle.

6. **Body Image:** Yoga promotes a positive body image by encouraging women to cultivate a loving and respectful relationship with their bodies. Yoga practices focus on body awareness, acceptance, and appreciation, helping women connect with their bodies in a supportive and empowering way.

7. **Resilience:** Yoga builds resilience by helping women develop mental and emotional strength, flexibility, and adaptability in the face of life's challenges. Through yoga, women learn to cultivate resilience by facing difficulties with courage, perseverance, and an open heart.

8. **Connection and Support:** Yoga communities provide women with a supportive and nurturing environment where they can connect with like-minded individuals, share experiences, and receive encouragement and guidance on their wellness journey. Building connections and receiving support from others can be incredibly validating and empowering for women's mental health and emotional well-being.

Overall, yoga offers women a holistic approach to mental health and emotional well-being, providing practices and tools that support self-care, healing, and personal growth. By incorporating yoga into their lives, women can cultivate greater resilience, balance, and vitality, allowing them to thrive in all aspects of their lives.

# CHAPTER SIX

## ADVANCED YOGA PRACTICES

Advanced yoga practices go beyond the basics, challenging practitioners both physically and mentally while deepening their connection to themselves and the practice. Here are some advanced yoga practices to explore:

1. **Advanced Asanas:** Advanced yoga poses require strength, flexibility, and balance. Poses such as Handstand (Adho Mukha Vrksasana), Forearm Stand (Pincha Mayurasana), and Scorpion Pose (Vrischikasana) challenge practitioners to refine their alignment, focus, and breath control while building physical prowess.

2. **Pranayama:** Advanced pranayama techniques involve intricate breath control to balance and energize the body and mind. Practices such as Kapalabhati (Skull Shining Breath), Bhastrika (Bellows Breath), and Nadi Shodhana (Alternate Nostril Breathing) require concentration, precision, and mastery of the breath.

3. **Bandhas:** Bandhas are energetic locks that help control the flow of prana (life force energy) within the body. Advanced practitioners learn to engage and release the three main bandhas—the Mula Bandha (Root Lock), Uddiyana Bandha

(Abdominal Lock), and Jalandhara Bandha (Throat Lock)—to enhance stability, strength, and energetic awareness in their practice.

4. **Meditation:** Advanced meditation practices deepen the practitioner's ability to focus, quiet the mind, and cultivate inner stillness and clarity. Techniques such as Vipassana (Insight Meditation), Metta (Loving-Kindness Meditation), and Dhyana (Deep Meditation) help advanced practitioners access higher states of consciousness and spiritual insight.

5. **Yoga Philosophy:** Advanced practitioners delve deeper into the philosophical underpinnings of yoga, studying ancient texts such as the Yoga Sutras of Patanjali, the Bhagavad Gita, and the Hatha Yoga Pradipika. They explore concepts such as the eight limbs of yoga, karma (action), dharma (duty), and self-realization (Atma Jnana).

6. **Sequencing and Creative Expression:** Advanced practitioners have the knowledge and skill to craft intricate and creative yoga sequences that challenge the body, mind, and spirit. They may incorporate elements of flow, inversions, arm balances, and backbends into their sequences, creating a dynamic and transformative experience for themselves and their students.

7. **Yoga Nidra:** Yoga Nidra, or yogic sleep, is a powerful guided meditation practice that induces

deep relaxation and rejuvenation. Advanced practitioners can guide themselves and others through the stages of Yoga Nidra, accessing states of deep rest, healing, and inner transformation.

8. **Yoga Therapy:** Advanced practitioners may explore the therapeutic applications of yoga, using specific techniques and practices to address physical, mental, and emotional imbalances. They may specialize in areas such as trauma-sensitive yoga, yoga for chronic pain management, or yoga for mental health and well-being.

Advanced yoga practices require dedication, discipline, and a willingness to explore the depths of the practice. They offer opportunities for growth, transformation, and self-discovery, empowering practitioners to embody the full potential of yoga in their lives.

## MASTERING ADVANCED PRACTICE AND TRANSITIONS

Mastering advanced yoga practice and transitions requires dedication, patience, and a deep understanding of both the physical and subtle aspects of the practice. Here are some tips to help you progress in your advanced yoga practice:

1. **Build a Strong Foundation:** Before attempting advanced poses and transitions, ensure

you have a solid foundation in the basics of yoga, including proper alignment, breath control, and body awareness. Regular practice of foundational poses will help you develop the strength, flexibility, and stability needed for advanced practice.

2. **Work with a Qualified Teacher:** Advanced yoga poses and transitions can be challenging and potentially risky if not practiced mindfully and with proper alignment. Work with a qualified yoga teacher who can offer guidance, support, and feedback to help you progress safely and effectively in your practice.

3. **Break Down Complex Movements:** Break down advanced poses and transitions into smaller, more manageable parts. Practice individual components of the pose or transition, focusing on proper alignment, engagement, and breath control. Gradually build up to the full expression of the pose or transition as you feel ready.

4. **Use Props and Modifications:** Props such as blocks, straps, and bolsters can provide support and assistance as you work on advanced poses and transitions. Don't be afraid to use props and modifications to help you access the pose safely and effectively, especially if you're working on challenging transitions or recovering from an injury.

5. **Develop Mindfulness and Concentration:** Advanced yoga practice requires a high level of

mindfulness and concentration. Cultivate present-moment awareness and focus on the sensations in your body as you move through poses and transitions. Tune into your breath and use it as a guide to help you move with intention and awareness.

6. **Practice Patience and Persistence:** Mastering advanced yoga poses and transitions takes time, patience, and consistent practice. Be patient with yourself and trust the process of growth and transformation in your practice. Celebrate progress, no matter how small, and stay committed to your practice even when faced with challenges or setbacks.

7. **Listen to Your Body:** Pay attention to your body's signals and honor its limitations. Respect any pain or discomfort you may experience and avoid pushing yourself beyond your edge. Be mindful of any existing injuries or conditions and modify your practice as needed to ensure safety and well-being.

8. **Seek Inspiration and Exploration:** Draw inspiration from experienced yogis and explore different styles and approaches to advanced yoga practice. Attend workshops, retreats, and classes led by seasoned teachers who can offer new insights, techniques, and perspectives to enrich your practice.

By following these tips and approaching your advanced yoga practice with humility, curiosity, and dedication, you can progress steadily and confidently towards mastering advanced poses and transitions, deepening your understanding of yoga, and experiencing the transformative power of the practice.

# EXPLORING PRANAYAMA AND MEDITATION OF A DEEPER LEVEL

Exploring pranayama (breath control) and meditation on a deeper level can lead to profound insights, inner transformation, and a greater sense of connection with oneself and the world around you. Here are some ways to deepen your practice of pranayama and meditation:

1. **Steady and Consistent Practice:** Consistency is key to deepening your practice of pranayama and meditation. Set aside time each day for dedicated practice, even if it's just a few minutes. Over time, regular practice will help you develop greater focus, awareness, and sensitivity to the subtle aspects of your breath and mind.

2. **Exploration of Different Techniques:** There are many different techniques of pranayama and meditation, each offering unique benefits and effects on the body and mind. Experiment with various techniques such as Ujjayi breath, Nadi

Shodhana (alternate nostril breathing), Kapalabhati (skull-shining breath), and Bhramari (bee breath) to discover which practices resonate most deeply with you.

**3. **Guided Practice and Instruction:**** Seek out guidance and instruction from experienced teachers or resources such as books, videos, or online courses to deepen your understanding and practice of pranayama and meditation. A knowledgeable teacher can offer valuable insights, corrections, and support as you explore these practices.

**4. **Integration with Asana Practice:**** Integrate pranayama and meditation into your yoga asana practice to create a more holistic and integrated experience. Use breath awareness and mindfulness techniques to deepen your presence and connection with each movement and posture.

**5. **Exploration of Subtle Energy:**** Pranayama and meditation offer a gateway to exploring the subtle energy body, including the flow of prana (life force energy) through the nadis (energy channels) and chakras (energy centers). Cultivate awareness of the subtle sensations and energetic shifts that arise during your practice, and explore techniques such as Bhuta Shuddhi (elemental purification) to balance and harmonize the energy body.

6. **Mindfulness in Daily Life:** Bring the principles of pranayama and meditation into your daily life by practicing mindfulness and presence in everyday activities. Cultivate awareness of your breath, thoughts, and emotions as you go about your day, and use breath awareness and mindfulness techniques to stay grounded and centered amidst the busyness of life.

7. **Self-Inquiry and Reflection:** Use pranayama and meditation as tools for self-inquiry and introspection. Explore questions such as "Who am I?" and "What is the nature of reality?" through contemplative practices such as Jnana Yoga (the yoga of wisdom) and self-reflection. Cultivate a sense of curiosity, openness, and humility as you explore these deeper existential questions.

8. **Satsang and Community Support:** Seek out community and support from like-minded practitioners through satsang (spiritual gatherings), meditation groups, or online forums. Sharing experiences, insights, and challenges with others on the spiritual path can offer valuable support and encouragement on your journey of self-discovery and transformation.

By approaching pranayama and meditation with dedication, curiosity, and an open heart, you can deepen your practice and experience profound states of inner peace, clarity, and connection with the divine within and around you.

# INCORPORATING YOGA PHILOSOPHY INTO DAILY LIFE

Incorporating yoga philosophy into daily life is a transformative practice that can enrich your experience, cultivate inner peace, and enhance your connection with yourself and the world around you. Here are some practical ways to integrate yoga philosophy into your everyday life:

1. **Mindfulness and Presence:** Practice mindfulness and presence in your daily activities by bringing your awareness to the present moment. Cultivate mindfulness while eating, walking, working, or engaging in any daily task, allowing yourself to fully immerse in the experience without judgment or distraction.

2. **Living with Ahimsa (Non-Violence):** Embody the principle of ahimsa (non-violence) by practicing kindness, compassion, and empathy towards yourself and others. Be mindful of your thoughts, words, and actions, and strive to act with kindness and consideration in all your interactions.

3. **Practicing Gratitude:** Cultivate gratitude for the blessings and abundance in your life by practicing gratitude rituals such as keeping a gratitude journal, expressing thanks to loved ones, or offering prayers of gratitude before meals.

Recognize and appreciate the beauty and wonder of life's simple pleasures.

4. **Santosha (Contentment):** Cultivate contentment and acceptance of what is by embracing the present moment with an open heart and mind. Practice gratitude for what you have rather than focusing on what you lack, and find joy and fulfillment in the simple pleasures of life.

5. **Self-Study (Svadhyaya):** Engage in self-study and self-reflection to deepen your understanding of yourself and your place in the world. Explore yoga philosophy through reading sacred texts such as the Bhagavad Gita, the Yoga Sutras of Patanjali, or the Upanishads, and reflect on how their teachings apply to your life.

6. **Seva (Selfless Service):** Practice seva, or selfless service, by offering your time, skills, and resources to serve others in need. Volunteer for charitable organizations, offer support to friends or family members in need, or engage in acts of kindness and compassion in your community.

7. **Mindful Communication:** Practice mindful communication by speaking with honesty, integrity, and compassion. Listen deeply to others with an open heart and mind, and communicate with kindness, respect, and empathy in all your interactions.

8. **Dedicated Spiritual Practice:** Establish a dedicated spiritual practice that includes yoga, meditation, pranayama, and self-reflection. Set aside time each day for practice, even if it's just a few minutes, and commit to nurturing your spiritual growth and evolution.

9. **Integration of Asana Practice:** Bring the principles of yoga philosophy into your asana practice by infusing each posture with intention, mindfulness, and awareness. Use your practice as an opportunity for self-inquiry, self-expression, and spiritual exploration.

10. **Connection with Nature:** Cultivate a deep connection with nature by spending time outdoors, immersing yourself in the beauty and tranquility of the natural world. Practice mindfulness in nature, observe the interconnectedness of all living beings, and find solace and inspiration in the rhythms of the earth.

By incorporating these principles of yoga philosophy into your daily life, you can cultivate greater peace, harmony, and fulfillment, and live with greater alignment with your true nature and purpose.

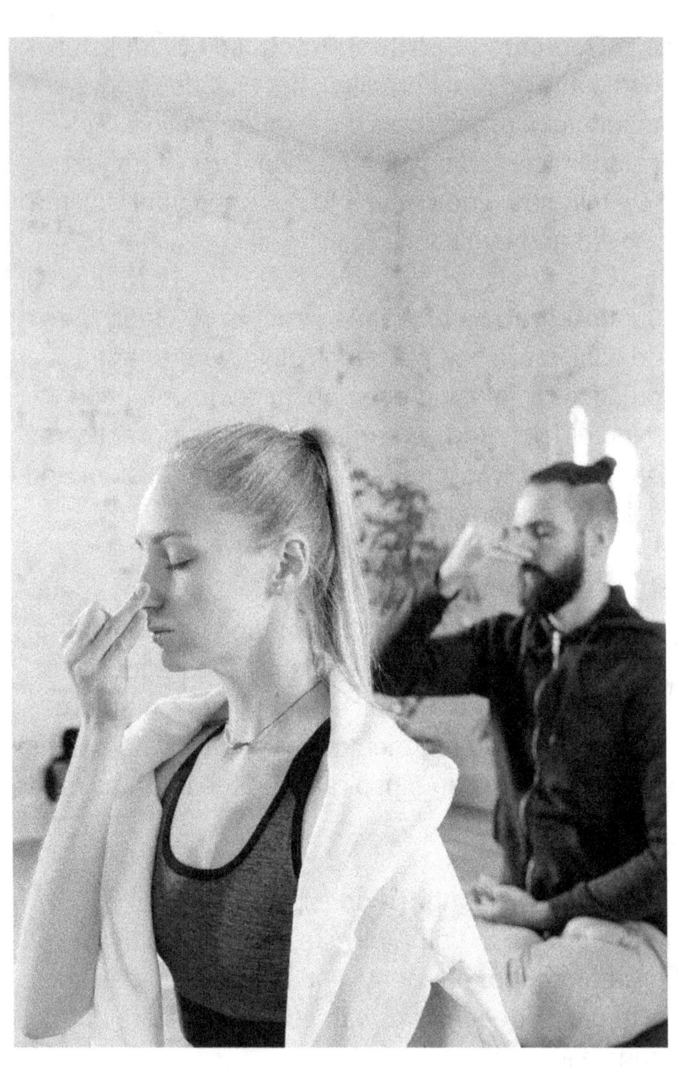

# CHAPTER SEVEN

## YOGA FOR SPECIFIC WOMEN'S CONCERN

The following are yoga for specific women's concern:

## YOGA FOR MENOPAUSE SYMPTOMS

Yoga can be a valuable tool for managing the symptoms of menopause, offering relief from physical discomfort, emotional fluctuations, and stress. Here are some ways yoga can help alleviate menopause symptoms:

1. **Hot Flashes and Night Sweats:** Gentle yoga poses and breathwork can help regulate body temperature and reduce the frequency and intensity of hot flashes and night sweats. Cooling poses such as Legs-Up-the-Wall Pose, Supported Bridge Pose, and Seated Forward Bend can help soothe the nervous system and calm the body's response to heat.

2. **Mood Swings and Emotional Instability:** Yoga can help stabilize mood and promote emotional well-being by balancing the nervous system and calming the mind. Practices such as gentle yoga, restorative yoga, and yoga nidra (yogic sleep) can help reduce stress, anxiety, and

irritability, fostering a greater sense of peace and equanimity.

3. **Insomnia and Sleep Disturbances:** Yoga can promote restful sleep and alleviate insomnia by calming the mind and relaxing the body. Practices such as gentle stretching, restorative poses, and relaxation techniques can help prepare the body for sleep and improve sleep quality.

4. **Joint Pain and Muscle Stiffness:** Yoga poses that focus on gentle stretching and strengthening can help relieve joint pain and muscle stiffness associated with menopause. Poses such as Cat-Cow Pose, Child's Pose, and Gentle Twists can help increase flexibility, reduce tension, and improve range of motion in the joints.

5. **Bone Health:** Weight-bearing yoga poses help strengthen the bones and reduce the risk of osteoporosis, a common concern for women during menopause. Poses such as Warrior II, Triangle Pose, and Chair Pose can help build bone density and improve overall bone health.

6. **Stress Reduction:** Yoga offers effective tools for managing stress and promoting relaxation, which can be particularly beneficial during the menopausal transition. Mindfulness practices, breathing techniques, and meditation can help calm the nervous system, reduce cortisol levels, and promote a sense of calm and well-being.

7. **Hormonal Balance:** Certain yoga practices, such as inverted poses and pranayama (breathwork), can help balance hormone levels and support overall hormonal health. Practices such as Shoulder Stand, Legs-Up-the-Wall Pose, and Alternate Nostril Breathing can help regulate the endocrine system and promote hormonal balance.

8. **Self-Care and Self-Compassion:** Menopause is a significant life transition that can bring about physical and emotional changes. Yoga provides an opportunity for women to practice self-care and self-compassion, nurturing themselves through gentle movement, mindful breathing, and relaxation practices.

By incorporating yoga into their daily routine, women experiencing menopause can find relief from symptoms, support their overall health and well-being, and navigate this transformative phase of life with greater ease and resilience. It's important to listen to your body, honor its needs, and consult with a healthcare provider if you have any concerns or underlying health conditions.

## YOGA FOR PELVIC FLOOR HEALTH AND INCONTINENCE

Yoga can be a beneficial practice for pelvic floor health and incontinence, as it helps strengthen and tone the pelvic floor muscles, improve circulation, and increase awareness of the pelvic region. Here are some yoga practices specifically targeted for pelvic floor health:

1. **Pelvic Floor Awareness:** Begin by developing awareness of your pelvic floor muscles. Sit comfortably and gently engage the muscles of the pelvic floor by imagining lifting and drawing them inward. Avoid gripping or tensing other muscles in the abdomen, buttocks, or thighs.

2. **Pelvic Tilts:** Practice pelvic tilts to mobilize and strengthen the pelvic floor muscles. Lie on your back with knees bent and feet hip-width apart. Inhale to tilt your pelvis forward, arching your lower back slightly. Exhale to tilt your pelvis back, pressing your lower back into the floor. Repeat for several rounds, coordinating the movement with your breath.

3. **Bridge Pose (Setu Bandhasana):** Bridge pose strengthens the pelvic floor muscles, glutes, and hamstrings. Lie on your back with knees bent and feet hip-width apart. Inhale to lift your hips towards the ceiling, pressing into your feet and engaging your glutes and pelvic floor. Hold for a few breaths, then exhale to lower back down. Repeat for several rounds.

4. **Squat Pose (Malasana):** Squatting helps release tension in the pelvic floor and promotes

circulation to the pelvic organs. Stand with feet wider than hip-width apart, toes turned out slightly. Lower into a squat position, bringing your buttocks towards the floor while keeping your heels grounded. Bring your hands to prayer at your heart center to help balance. Hold for several breaths, then rise back up. .

5. **Pelvic Floor Breathing:** Practice deep diaphragmatic breathing while focusing on the pelvic floor muscles. Inhale deeply, allowing the belly and pelvic floor to relax and expand. Exhale fully, gently engaging the pelvic floor muscles as if lifting them upward. Repeat for several breaths, coordinating the movement with your breath.

6. **Cat-Cow Pose (Marjaryasana-Bitilasana):** Cat-Cow pose helps mobilize and strengthen the pelvic floor muscles while also improving spinal flexibility. Start on your hands and knees, with wrists aligned under shoulders and knees under hips. Inhale to arch your back and lift your tailbone and chest towards the ceiling (Cow Pose). Exhale to round your spine and tuck your chin towards your chest (Cat Pose). Flow between the two poses, coordinating movement with breath.

7. **Pelvic Floor Relaxation:** Practice deep relaxation techniques to release tension in the pelvic floor muscles. Lie on your back in Savasana (Corpse Pose) with legs extended and arms relaxed by your sides. Close your eyes and bring

awareness to your pelvic floor. Inhale deeply, allowing the pelvic floor to relax and soften. Exhale fully, releasing any tension or tightness. Repeat for several minutes, allowing the entire body to relax deeply.

Regular practice of these yoga poses and techniques can help improve pelvic floor strength, tone, and function, reducing symptoms of incontinence and promoting overall pelvic health. It's important to listen to your body, practice mindfully, and consult with a healthcare provider if you have any concerns or underlying health conditions.

## YOGA FOR BREAST CANCER SURVIVORS AND RECOVERY

Yoga can play a valuable role in the recovery and rehabilitation process for breast cancer survivors, offering physical, emotional, and spiritual support throughout the journey. Here are some ways yoga can benefit breast cancer survivors:

1. **Physical Healing:** Gentle yoga poses and movements can help improve flexibility, strength, and range of motion in the body, especially areas affected by surgery or treatment such as the chest, shoulders, and arms. Yoga poses such as gentle stretches, chest openers, and shoulder rotations

can help alleviate tightness, reduce scar tissue, and promote healing.

2. **Lymphatic Health:** Yoga practices that incorporate gentle movements and breathwork can help support lymphatic circulation, which is important for reducing swelling, promoting detoxification, and maintaining immune function. Practices such as gentle twisting poses, lymphatic massage techniques, and diaphragmatic breathing can help stimulate lymphatic flow and support overall lymphatic health.

3. **Stress Reduction:** Yoga offers effective tools for managing stress, anxiety, and emotional distress, which are common concerns for breast cancer survivors. Mindfulness practices such as meditation, deep breathing, and guided relaxation can help calm the nervous system, reduce cortisol levels, and promote a sense of peace and well-being.

4. **Fatigue Management:** Fatigue is a common side effect of cancer treatment, and yoga can help alleviate fatigue by promoting relaxation, restorative rest, and gentle movement. Practices such as restorative yoga, yoga nidra (yogic sleep), and gentle breathing techniques can help restore energy levels, improve sleep quality, and enhance overall vitality.

5. **Body Image and Self-Esteem:** Breast cancer treatment can have profound effects on body image and self-esteem, and yoga offers a safe and supportive space for survivors to reconnect with their bodies, cultivate self-compassion, and foster a sense of acceptance and empowerment. Gentle yoga poses, meditation, and self-reflection practices can help survivors navigate feelings of loss, grief, and change, and embrace their bodies with love and gratitude.

6. **Community and Support:** Participating in yoga classes or support groups specifically for breast cancer survivors can provide valuable community, connection, and support. Sharing experiences, insights, and challenges with others who have gone through similar experiences can offer validation, encouragement, and a sense of belonging on the healing journey.

7. **Empowerment and Resilience:** Yoga teaches valuable life skills such as mindfulness, resilience, and self-awareness, which can support survivors in navigating the challenges and uncertainties of life after cancer. By cultivating inner strength, courage, and adaptability through yoga practice, survivors can embrace their journey with greater confidence, grace, and resilience.

It's important for breast cancer survivors to approach yoga practice with sensitivity to their individual needs, limitations, and preferences.

Consulting with a qualified yoga teacher or healthcare provider can help survivors tailor their yoga practice to suit their unique circumstances and support their ongoing recovery and well-being.

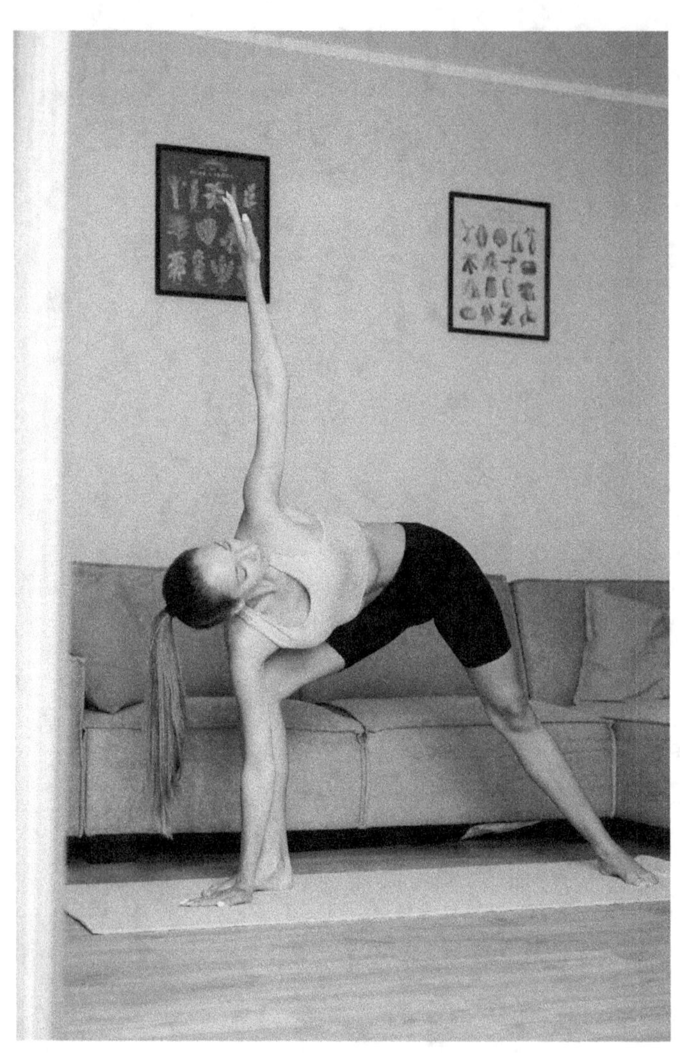

# CHAPTER EIGHT

## PARTNER AND GROUP YOGA FOR CONNECTION

Partner and group yoga can be a wonderful way to deepen connections, build trust, and cultivate a sense of community among participants. Here are some partner and group yoga poses and activities to foster connection:

1. **Partner Yoga Poses:**
   - **Partner Forward Fold:** Sit back-to-back with your partner, legs extended. Lean forward simultaneously, folding over your legs, and reach for each other's hands.
   - **Partner Tree Pose:** Stand side by side with your partner, holding hands. Lift one foot and place the sole against the inner thigh of the opposite leg. Find your balance together.
   - **Partner Seated Twist:** Sit facing each other with legs crossed. Hold onto each other's opposite knee and twist towards the side, mirroring each other's movement.

2. **Group Yoga Poses and Activities:**
   - **Circle of Asanas:** Stand in a circle and take turns leading the group through a series of yoga poses. Each participant can add their own creative variations.

- **Group Sun Salutation:** Perform a synchronized Sun Salutation sequence together as a group, coordinating movement and breath.
   - **Partner Massage Train:** Sit in a line with one person behind the other. The person in front leans forward, while the person behind gently massages their shoulders. Continue the chain down the line.

3. **Partner and Group Breathing Exercises:**
   - **Synchronized Breathing:** Sit facing each other, close your eyes, and synchronize your breath. Inhale deeply together, then exhale completely. Focus on the rhythm of your breath and the connection with your partner or group.
   - **Group Om Chanting:** Sit or stand in a circle and chant "Om" together as a group. Feel the vibrations resonate through your body and connect with the collective energy of the group.

4. **Partner and Group Relaxation:**
   - **Partner Savasana:** Lie down next to your partner, with your heads towards each other. Place one hand on your partner's heart and one hand on their belly, and vice versa. Close your eyes and breathe together, allowing both bodies to relax deeply.
   - **Group Meditation:** Sit in a circle and lead the group through a guided meditation or visualization practice focused on connection, compassion, and unity.

**5. **Partner and Group Trust-Building Activities:****

- ****Partner Trust Falls:**** Stand facing away from your partner, arms crossed over your chest. Lean back slowly and trust your partner to catch you.

- ****Group Trust Circles:**** Stand in a circle with arms extended to the sides, palms facing up. Lean back and allow yourself to be supported by the group, creating a sense of trust and unity.

These partner and group yoga poses and activities can help foster connection, communication, and trust among participants, creating a supportive and uplifting environment for practicing yoga together. Remember to approach these practices with openness, respect, and a spirit of collaboration.

# EXPLORING PARTNER YOGA POSES AND PRACTICES

Exploring partner yoga poses and practices can be a fun and rewarding way to deepen your connection with a friend, partner, or loved one while enhancing your yoga practice. Here are some partner yoga poses and practices to try:

**1. **Double Downward Dog:**** Start in Downward Dog pose facing your partner, with some distance between you. Both partners walk their hands forward, lowering their chests towards the ground while keeping their hips high. Hold hands with your partner and press into your palms to deepen the stretch.

2. **Seated Spinal Twist:** Sit facing your partner with your legs crossed. Hold hands with your partner and lengthen your spines. Inhale to lengthen, and exhale to twist gently to one side, while your partner twists in the opposite direction. Use your partner's hands for support and deepen the twist with each exhale.

3. **Back-to-Back Chair Pose:** Stand back-to-back with your partner, with your feet hip-width apart. Lean against each other for support as you bend your knees and lower into Chair Pose. Press your backs against each other for added stability and hold the pose for several breaths.

4. **Flying High:** Partner 1 stands with feet hip-width apart, while Partner 2 stands facing them, holding onto Partner 1's forearms. Partner 1 leans forward slightly, and Partner 2 lifts their legs off the ground, extending them straight back behind them. Partner 1 supports Partner 2's legs while keeping their core engaged.

5. **Partner Boat Pose:** Sit facing each other with your knees bent and feet flat on the ground. Hold hands with your partner and lean back slightly, engaging your core muscles. Lift your feet off the ground, bringing your shins parallel to the floor.

Find your balance together and hold the pose while maintaining eye contact.

6. **Double Plank:** Partner 1 starts in Plank Pose, while Partner 2 stands behind them, facing their feet. Partner 2 carefully steps onto Partner 1's back, placing their hands on Partner 1's shoulders for support. Both partners engage their core muscles and hold the pose for several breaths.

7. **Partner Tree Pose:** Stand side by side with your partner, holding hands for balance. Shift your weight onto one foot and place the sole of your other foot against the inner thigh of your standing leg. Your partner mirrors your movements, pressing their foot against the opposite leg. Find your balance together and extend your arms overhead.

8. **Partner Forward Fold:** Stand facing your partner with your feet hip-width apart. Hold hands with your partner and walk back slightly, creating a slight tension in your arms. On an exhale, both partners hinge forward at the hips, folding forward together. Keep a slight bend in your knees and allow your spine to lengthen as you fold forward.

Remember to communicate with your partner throughout the practice, listen to your body, and modify poses as needed to ensure safety and comfort. Partner yoga is not only a physical practice but also an opportunity to deepen trust, communication, and connection with your partner.

Enjoy the journey of exploration and discovery together!

## BUILDING TRUST AND CONNECTION THROUGH YOGA WITH FRIENDS AND FAMILY

Building trust and connection through yoga with friends and family can be a beautiful way to deepen your relationships and create meaningful experiences together. Here are some tips for fostering trust and connection through yoga:

1. **Practice Active Listening:** Before beginning your yoga practice, take a few moments to check in with each other and share any intentions or concerns you may have. Practice active listening by giving each person the opportunity to express themselves without interruption or judgment.

2. **Set Intentions Together:** Set intentions or themes for your yoga practice as a group, such as gratitude, compassion, or presence. Aligning your intentions can create a sense of unity and shared purpose, deepening your connection with each other and the practice.

3. **Create a Safe Space:** Establish a safe and supportive environment for your yoga practice, free from judgment or competition. Encourage each person to honor their own boundaries and listen to

their body's signals, emphasizing self-care and self-compassion throughout the practice.

4. **Practice Partner Yoga:** Explore partner yoga poses and practices that require trust, communication, and collaboration. Partner poses such as Double Downward Dog, Partner Boat Pose, and Flying High can foster a sense of connection and mutual support as you work together in tandem.

5. **Offer Hands-On Support:** Offer hands-on assistance and support to each other during yoga poses, providing gentle adjustments or assists as needed. Use mindful touch to offer encouragement, stability, and alignment, fostering a deeper sense of connection and trust between partners.

6. **Encourage Vulnerability:** Encourage each person to be vulnerable and authentic in their practice, allowing themselves to fully experience and express their thoughts, emotions, and sensations. Create a non-judgmental space where everyone feels accepted and supported in their journey.

7. **Practice Partner Breathing:** Explore synchronized breathing exercises with your partner or group, such as mirroring each other's breath or practicing deep belly breathing together. Shared breathwork can foster a sense of connection and

harmony, aligning your energy and intentions as a group.

8. **Reflect and Share:** After your yoga practice, take time to reflect and share your experiences with each other. Discuss what insights or feelings arose during the practice and how it impacted your sense of connection and trust with each other.

9. **Express Gratitude:** End your yoga practice with a gratitude circle, where each person has the opportunity to express appreciation for themselves and each other. Reflect on the support and connection you've experienced during the practice and acknowledge the bonds of friendship and love that unite you.

By incorporating these practices into your yoga sessions with friends and family, you can create a nurturing and empowering space for building trust, connection, and mutual support, both on and off the mat. Enjoy the journey of deepening your relationships through the transformative power of yoga!

## YOGA RETREATS AND WORKSHOPS FOR WOMEN

Yoga retreats and workshops specifically designed for women offer a unique opportunity for self-discovery, rejuvenation, and connection with other like-minded individuals. Here's what you can expect from attending a yoga retreat or workshop tailored for women:

1. **Empowerment and Inspiration:** Women's yoga retreats and workshops often focus on empowering women to embrace their unique strengths, cultivate self-confidence, and awaken their inner wisdom. Through inspiring teachings, guided practices, and interactive workshops, participants are encouraged to tap into their full potential and live authentically.

2. **Supportive Community:** These retreats provide a supportive and nurturing environment where women can come together to share experiences, insights, and challenges in a safe and non-judgmental space. Building connections with other women who share similar interests and aspirations can be incredibly empowering and uplifting.

3. **Holistic Well-being:** Women's yoga retreats typically offer a holistic approach to well-being, addressing not only the physical aspects of yoga but also mental, emotional, and spiritual aspects. Participants may engage in a variety of practices such as yoga asana, meditation, pranayama, self-reflection, and mindfulness to promote balance and harmony in all areas of their lives.

4. **Self-care and Relaxation:** Retreats provide an opportunity for women to prioritize self-care and relaxation, away from the demands and stresses of everyday life. Participants can indulge in nourishing activities such as massage, spa treatments, nature walks, and healthy meals, allowing them to unwind and rejuvenate body, mind, and spirit.

5. **Exploration and Growth:** Women's retreats often include workshops and activities designed to facilitate personal growth, self-discovery, and transformation. Participants may explore topics such as women's health and wellness, body image, relationships, sexuality, creativity, and life purpose, gaining valuable insights and tools for living a fulfilling and meaningful life.

6. **Celebration of Feminine Energy:** These retreats celebrate the beauty and power of feminine energy, honoring the unique gifts and strengths that women bring to the world. Through rituals, ceremonies, and sacred practices, participants can reconnect with their feminine essence and embrace their innate wisdom, intuition, and creativity.

7. **Expert Guidance and Support:** Retreats are typically led by experienced yoga teachers, wellness practitioners, and facilitators who specialize in women's health and empowerment. These experts provide guidance, support, and inspiration throughout the retreat, offering

personalized attention and encouragement to each
participant.

**8. **Transformative Experience:**** Attending a
women's yoga retreat or workshop can be a
transformative experience, leaving participants
feeling inspired, rejuvenated, and empowered to
live their best lives. The supportive community,
nurturing environment, and transformative practices
offered at these retreats can catalyze profound
shifts and lasting positive changes in participants'
lives.

Whether you're looking to deepen your yoga
practice, connect with other women, or simply take
a break and recharge, a women's yoga retreat or
workshop can offer a transformative and
empowering experience that nourishes body, mind,
and soul.

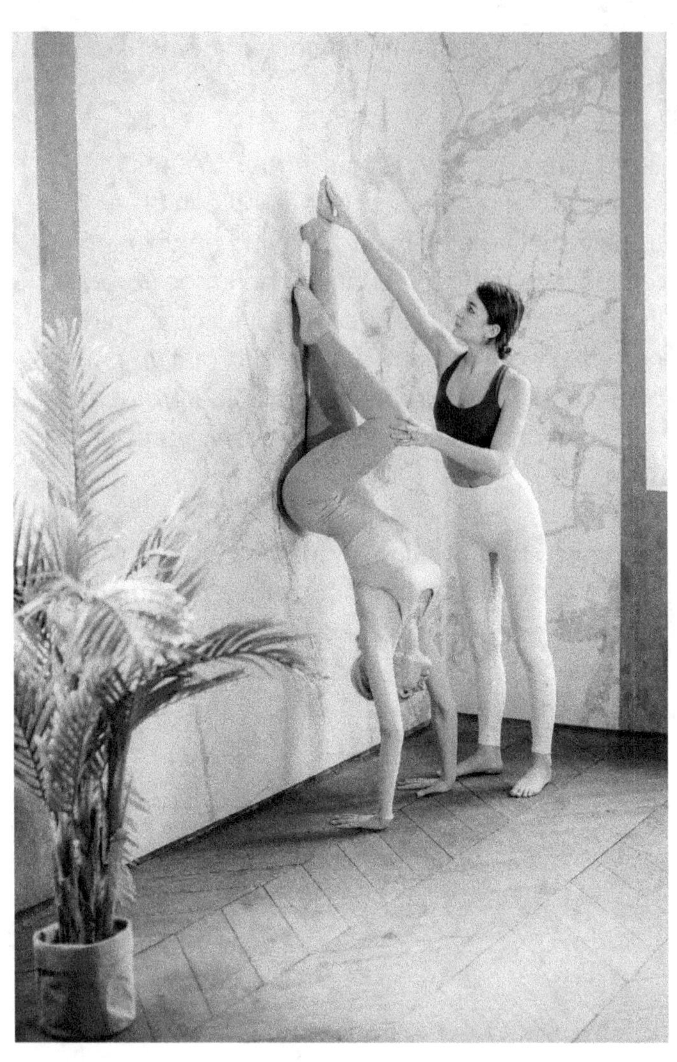

# CHAPTER NINE

## YOGA LIFESTYLE AND SAFE-CARE

Living a yoga lifestyle encompasses more than just practicing yoga on the mat; it's about incorporating the principles of yoga into every aspect of your life, promoting holistic well-being, and fostering a sense of balance, harmony, and connection with yourself and the world around you. Here are some key components of a yoga lifestyle and tips for practicing safe self-care:

1. **Yoga Practice:** Dedicate time each day for yoga practice, whether it's asana (physical postures), pranayama (breathwork), meditation, or self-reflection. Listen to your body and practice with awareness, honoring your limitations and avoiding pushing yourself into pain or discomfort.

2. **Healthy Eating:** Nourish your body with wholesome, nutritious foods that support your overall health and well-being. Eat mindfully, savoring each bite and paying attention to how different foods make you feel. Prioritize whole grains, fruits, vegetables, lean proteins, and healthy fats, and minimize processed foods and added sugars.

3. **Self-Care Practices:** Prioritize self-care and make time for activities that nourish your body, mind, and soul. This can include activities such as journaling, spending time in nature, taking relaxing baths, practicing gratitude, and engaging in creative pursuits that bring you joy.

4. **Mindfulness and Presence:** Cultivate mindfulness and presence in your daily life by bringing your attention to the present moment. Practice mindfulness in everyday activities such as eating, walking, and interacting with others, noticing sensations, thoughts, and emotions without judgment.

5. **Connection and Community:** Cultivate meaningful connections with others and foster a sense of community and support. Spend time with loved ones, engage in activities that bring you closer to others, and seek out like-minded individuals who share your values and interests.

6. **Sustainable Living:** Practice ahimsa (non-violence) towards the environment by adopting sustainable and eco-friendly lifestyle practices. Reduce your carbon footprint, minimize waste, and make choices that promote environmental conservation and stewardship.

7. **Rest and Relaxation:** Prioritize rest and relaxation to recharge your body and mind. Get enough sleep each night, aim for at least 7-8 hours

of quality sleep, and create a calming bedtime routine to promote relaxation and restful sleep.

8. **Emotional Well-being:** Take care of your emotional well-being by acknowledging and processing your feelings, practicing self-compassion, and seeking support when needed. Practice techniques such as deep breathing, meditation, and mindfulness to manage stress and promote emotional balance.

9. **Continued Learning:** Stay curious and open to learning, exploring new ideas, and expanding your knowledge of yoga and holistic health. Attend workshops, read books, listen to podcasts, and engage in continuing education opportunities to deepen your understanding and practice.

10. **Safe Practice:** Practice yoga safely by listening to your body, respecting your limits, and seeking guidance from qualified teachers or healthcare professionals when needed. Avoid pushing yourself into pain or discomfort, and honor your body's need for rest and recovery.

By incorporating these principles into your daily life and practicing safe self-care, you can cultivate a yoga lifestyle that promotes holistic well-being, resilience, and vitality, allowing you to live with greater joy, purpose, and fulfillment.

# INTEGRATING YOGA INTO DAILY LIFE FOR WOMEN

Integrating yoga into daily life for women is a wonderful way to cultivate balance, well-being, and resilience amidst the demands and challenges of modern life. Here are some practical tips for incorporating yoga into your daily routine:

1. **Morning Yoga Routine:** Start your day with a short yoga practice to energize your body and calm your mind. Even just 10-15 minutes of gentle stretching, sun salutations, and deep breathing can set a positive tone for the day ahead.

2. **Mindful Movement:** Infuse mindfulness into everyday activities such as walking, cooking, cleaning, and commuting. Pay attention to your breath, body sensations, and surroundings as you move through your daily tasks, turning mundane activities into opportunities for presence and awareness.

3. **Desk Yoga Breaks:** Take short yoga breaks throughout the day to release tension and recenter your mind and body. Incorporate simple stretches, seated twists, neck rolls, and deep breathing exercises into your workday to relieve stiffness and boost productivity.

4. **Yoga Nidra or Meditation:** Dedicate time each day for relaxation and stress relief through

practices such as yoga nidra (yogic sleep) or meditation. Set aside a few minutes during your lunch break or before bed to unwind, quiet your mind, and cultivate inner peace and calm.

5. **Yoga for Stress Management:** Use yoga as a tool for managing stress and promoting emotional well-being. Practice calming breathwork techniques such as alternate nostril breathing or belly breathing whenever you feel overwhelmed or anxious, and turn to restorative yoga poses to soothe frazzled nerves and restore balance.

6. **Yoga for Women's Health:** Tailor your yoga practice to support specific women's health needs, such as menstrual discomfort, hormonal balance, fertility, pregnancy, or menopause. Choose yoga poses and practices that address your unique concerns and promote overall health and vitality.

7. **Evening Wind-Down:** Wind down in the evening with a gentle yoga practice to relax your body and prepare for restful sleep. Focus on soothing, grounding poses such as forward folds, gentle twists, and restorative poses, accompanied by slow, deep breathing to signal to your body that it's time to unwind.

8. **Yoga with Friends or Family:** Share the benefits of yoga with friends or family members by practicing together. Organize weekly yoga sessions with loved ones, attend a yoga class together, or

explore partner yoga poses to deepen your connections and support each other's well-being.

9. **Gratitude and Reflection:** Take a few moments each day to cultivate gratitude and reflection through journaling or silent contemplation. Reflect on moments of joy, appreciation, and growth, and acknowledge the blessings in your life with a sense of gratitude and appreciation.

10. **Consistency and Adaptability:** Be consistent with your yoga practice while also remaining adaptable to life's fluctuations and changes. Be gentle with yourself on days when your energy levels are low or your schedule is busy, and adjust your practice accordingly to meet your needs in the present moment.

By integrating yoga into your daily life with intention and mindfulness, you can experience greater balance, resilience, and well-being, nurturing your body, mind, and spirit on and off the mat.

## CREATING A BALANCED YOGA ROUTINE

Creating a balanced yoga routine involves incorporating a variety of elements that address different aspects of physical, mental, and emotional well-being. Here's how you can create a well-rounded yoga practice:

1. **Warm-Up:** Start your practice with a gentle warm-up to prepare your body for movement. This can include gentle stretches, joint mobilization exercises, and dynamic movements to increase blood flow and flexibility.

2. **Asana (Physical Postures):** Include a mix of standing, seated, supine, and prone yoga poses to work all areas of the body. Focus on poses that strengthen, stretch, and balance different muscle groups, incorporating variations and modifications to suit your level and needs.

3. **Sun Salutations (Surya Namaskar):** Incorporate Sun Salutations into your practice to build heat, improve circulation, and increase flexibility. Sun Salutations provide a dynamic sequence that works the entire body and can serve as a foundation for your practice.

4. **Strength-Building Poses:** Include poses that target major muscle groups and promote strength and stability. Poses such as Warrior series, Chair Pose, Plank Pose, and Boat Pose are excellent for building strength in the legs, core, arms, and back.

5. **Flexibility and Stretching:** Incorporate poses that focus on stretching and lengthening muscles to improve flexibility and range of motion. Include forward folds, hip openers, backbends, and

twists to release tension and increase mobility in different areas of the body.

6. **Balance Poses:** Include balance poses to improve stability, focus, and concentration. Poses such as Tree Pose, Eagle Pose, and Half Moon Pose challenge your balance while also strengthening the muscles of the legs and core.

7. **Pranayama (Breathwork):** Integrate breathwork practices into your routine to enhance mindfulness, calm the nervous system, and deepen your connection with your breath. Explore techniques such as Ujjayi breath, Dirga breath, and Nadi Shodhana (alternate nostril breathing) to promote relaxation and focus.

8. **Meditation and Mindfulness:** Dedicate time for meditation and mindfulness practices to cultivate inner peace, clarity, and presence. Set aside a few minutes at the end of your practice for seated meditation or guided relaxation, allowing yourself to rest deeply and integrate the benefits of your practice.

9. **Cool Down and Relaxation:** Conclude your practice with a gentle cool down and relaxation sequence to release tension and promote relaxation. Include poses such as Child's Pose, Supine Twist, and Savasana (Corpse Pose) to unwind and surrender into stillness.

**10. **Self-Reflection:**** Take a few moments after your practice for self-reflection and gratitude. Acknowledge the effort you've put into your practice, notice any changes or insights that arise, and express gratitude for the opportunity to nourish your body, mind, and spirit through yoga.

By incorporating these elements into your yoga routine, you can create a balanced and holistic practice that supports your overall well-being and helps you cultivate strength, flexibility, balance, and inner peace both on and off the mat.

## PRACTICING SELF-CARE AND MINDFULNESS OFF THE MAT

Practicing self-care and mindfulness off the yoga mat is essential for maintaining balance, well-being, and inner peace in everyday life. Here are some ways to incorporate self-care and mindfulness into your daily routine:

**1. **Mindful Eating:**** Pay attention to your food choices and eating habits, savoring each bite and eating slowly with awareness. Notice the colors, textures, and flavors of your food, and listen to your body's hunger and fullness cues.

**2. **Daily Meditation:**** Dedicate time each day for meditation or mindfulness practice, even if it's just a few minutes. Find a quiet space where you can sit comfortably, close your eyes, and focus on your breath or a simple mantra. Allow thoughts to come and go without judgment, returning your attention to the present moment.

3. **Gratitude Practice:** Cultivate an attitude of gratitude by reflecting on the blessings and abundance in your life. Keep a gratitude journal and write down three things you're grateful for each day, whether it's a beautiful sunrise, a kind gesture from a friend, or a moment of peace and quiet.

4. **Digital Detox:** Take regular breaks from screens and technology to give your mind a rest and reconnect with the world around you. Set boundaries around device usage, such as turning off notifications during meal times or scheduling screen-free evenings for relaxation and quality time with loved ones.

5. **Nature Walks:** Spend time outdoors in nature, immersing yourself in the beauty and tranquility of the natural world. Take leisurely walks in the park, hike in the mountains, or simply sit and enjoy the sights and sounds of nature. Allow yourself to slow down and appreciate the present moment.

6. **Creative Expression:** Engage in creative activities that bring you joy and allow you to express yourself authentically. Whether it's painting,

writing, dancing, or playing music, find ways to tap into your creativity and nurture your soul.

7. **Self-Compassion:** Practice self-compassion and kindness towards yourself, especially during challenging times. Treat yourself with the same care and understanding you would offer to a dear friend, and be gentle with yourself when faced with setbacks or difficulties.

8. **Quality Sleep:** Prioritize quality sleep by establishing a consistent bedtime routine and creating a calming sleep environment. Aim for 7-9 hours of restful sleep each night, allowing your body and mind to recharge and rejuvenate for the day ahead.

9. **Connection with Others:** Cultivate meaningful connections with friends, family, and community members, nurturing supportive relationships that bring joy and fulfillment. Make time for regular social activities and heartfelt conversations, and offer support and compassion to those around you.

10. **Self-Reflection:** Take time for self-reflection and introspection, whether through journaling, contemplative walks, or quiet moments of solitude. Tune into your inner wisdom and intuition, and explore deeper aspects of yourself and your life's purpose.

By incorporating these practices into your daily life, you can cultivate a greater sense of well-being, resilience, and inner peace, fostering a harmonious relationship between mind, body, and spirit.

# CONCLUSION: EMBRACING YOUR YOGA JOURNEY AS A WOMAN

Embracing your yoga journey as a woman is a deeply personal and transformative experience that offers an opportunity for growth, self-discovery, and empowerment. As you embark on this journey, remember that yoga is not just a physical practice but a path to wholeness and well-being that encompasses all aspects of your being—body, mind, and spirit.

Throughout your yoga journey, you will encounter challenges and triumphs, moments of stillness and movement, and opportunities for self-reflection and growth. Embrace each step of the journey with an open heart and a curious mind, trusting in your innate wisdom and intuition to guide you along the way.

As a woman, your yoga practice can be a source of strength, resilience, and self-empowerment, helping you navigate the complexities of life with grace and compassion. Through yoga, you can cultivate a deeper connection to your body, honor your unique strengths and vulnerabilities, and reclaim your innate sense of worthiness and belonging.

As you continue on your yoga journey, remember
to:

1. **Listen to Your Body:** Honor your body's
wisdom and listen to its messages, respecting its
limits and boundaries while also challenging
yourself to grow and evolve.

2. **Cultivate Self-Compassion:** Be gentle with
yourself and practice self-compassion, especially
during times of difficulty or struggle. Treat yourself
with kindness, understanding, and love, knowing
that you are worthy of care and compassion.

3. **Trust Your Intuition:** Trust in your intuition and
inner guidance as you navigate your yoga practice
and life's journey. Tune into your inner wisdom and
let it be your compass, guiding you towards greater
authenticity and alignment with your true self.

4. **Celebrate Your Progress:** Celebrate your
progress and achievements, no matter how small
they may seem. Recognize the growth and
transformation that occur on your yoga journey and
celebrate the strength and resilience that you
embody as a woman.

5. **Connect with Community:** Seek out
community and support on your yoga journey,
surrounding yourself with like-minded individuals
who uplift and inspire you. Share your experiences,

insights, and challenges with others, knowing that you are not alone on this path.

6. **Embrace Imperfection:** Embrace imperfection and let go of the need for perfection in your yoga practice and in life. Embrace the journey itself, with all its twists and turns, knowing that it is through our imperfections that we find our greatest strength and beauty.

As you embrace your yoga journey as a woman, may you find joy, fulfillment, and deep connection with yourself and the world around you. May your practice be a source of inspiration, healing, and transformation, empowering you to live with courage, authenticity, and grace.

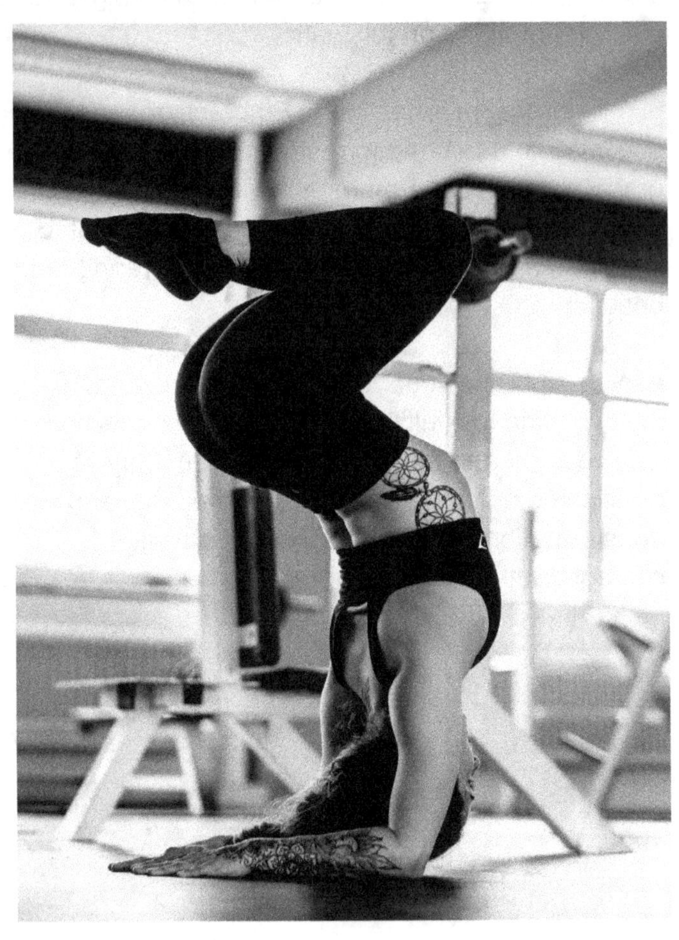